Praise for
The Handbook of Vintage Remedies

"Jessie Hawkins, MH suggests evidence-based, natural medical therapies that have been shown to be clinically effective alternative therapies. As an integrative family medicine physician, I am continually searching for sources of reliable medical information reporting on clinical applications of natural therapies. To that end, Ms. Hawkins' work makes an important contribution to educate everyone, families and health care providers, on clinical applications of proven therapies. Ms. Hawkins easily and respectfully negotiates the line between traditional and natural therapies and she understands the role that each can play in our health, and in how we choose to help our families lead healthy lives."

Daniel B. Kalb, MD, MPH, FAAFP

"Jessie Hawkin's passion and expertise are vast. She writes about health and herbal remedies in such a comforting and reassuring way."

Sara Snow; Green Lifestyle Expert, Author and TV Host

"Jessie has a knack for taking the mystery out of herbal use at home with the family. In her book, *The Handbook of Vintage Remedies,* she is effective in sharing the wisdom she has gleaned as an experienced mom and herbalist."

Susie Meeks, CPM-TN

"*The Handbook of Vintage Remedies* is a treasure chest of natural remedies for the home. Presented in a scientific, yet easy to understand way, herbalist Jessie Hawkins offers practical advice for all of us, mothers and professionals alike. This book is a must for any natural family!"

Daphne McIntosh CPM, LMT, RN, birth doula

"So many of my clients want to avoid the overuse of antibiotics and treat minor illnesses, aches and pains as naturally as possible. New moms looking for ways to use natural, herbal remedies for their families will find practical, easy-to-use information in Jessie's book,*The Handbook of Vintage Remedies*. It's on the 9 Months & Beyond, LLC recommended reading list!"

Micky Jones, BS, CLE, CLD, CHBE, HCHI, IBCLC

The Handbook of
VINTAGE REMEDIES

THE HANDBOOK OF VINTAGE REMEDIES
PUBLISHED BY THISTLE PUBLICATIONS
Spring Hill, Tennessee
a division of Vintage Remedies
www.VintageRemedies.com

ISBN 10: 0-9822318-5-7
ISBN 13: 978-0-9822318-5-2

Warning / Disclaimer: This book is intended as a reference volume only, not a medical manual. Every effort has been made to ensure that the information contained herein is complete and accurate. However, you should consult a physician, preferably a physician with experience in natural medicine before treating yourself with herbs or combining them with pharmaceuticals. Jessie Hawkins and Thistle Publications / Vintage Remedies shall have neither liability nor responsibility to any person or entity regarding any alleged loss, damage or injury as a result of the information presented in this work. Women who are pregnant, who may become pregnant, or are breastfeeding should not use herbs or any other medication without the approval of their primary care provider. If you suspect that you have a medical problem, please do not delay seeking competent help.

Hawkins, Jessie

The Handbook of Vintage Remedies / by Jessie Hawkins
-- 1st Edition

ISBN 10: 0-9822318-5-7

Printed in the United States of America
2008

To my amazing husband Matthew, to Grace, Joel and Micah, the three precious children I hold in my arms, and to Julia, the daughter in Ethiopia I long to hold.

To Jenny, who constantly reminded me how important this book was for mothers everywhere, encouraged me through the rough seasons in life, and continuously called to ask, "Is that book done, yet?!?" I miss you so much.

Contents

SECTION THREE: BOTANICAL APOTHECARY

ACKNOWLEDGMENTS

As I consider the nearly three years this book has been in the works, it seems impossible to recount and give proper thanks to everyone that has encouraged me along the way. From the first seedling of an idea, to the tireless nights and deadlines, and of course, the extended periods of time this book has been placed on the back burner to care for more immediate tasks, I have always known that this book is not my own. While my name graces the cover, there are many important individuals that played a role.

I must begin by thanking my Savior and my God, who saw it fit to create amazingly complex plants, and placed them here for our benefit as we journey through this world, and for the even greater miracle of choosing me as one of your own, though I am so far from deserving.

Next, comes my husband, Matthew, for your patience with me as I hurried through the end of yet another project, for your input (even when I didn't want to hear it!) and for your constant encouragement that Yes, someone would want to read my book!

I am so blessed to thank my sweet daughter Grace, who is bursting with ambition and passion that is continually inspiring, my meticulous son Joel, who brings me back to the center, encourages me to never stop learning, and teaches his mother patience, and my baby Micah, though you are not really a baby anymore, for your willingness to share your cuddly mommy with the laptop, and for teaching mommy perseverance. Of course, I cannot leave out my precious daughter Julia, who is somewhere in Ethiopia right now. Though I have yet to see you or hold you, I love you more than you can ever imagine.

My father, Joseph West, who sat with me every night of my childhood and read the Scriptures to me before bedtime. Those evenings will never be forgotten and have inspired in me a love for my Savior.

My dear friend Jenny, who encouraged me daily with your constant optimism, who continually reminded me that this book was important and that I was the herbalist to write it! Your cheerful voice on the other end of the phone is something I miss so much.

Thank you Lord for CeCe Lee, my priceless assistant, for working with my constantly multitasking brain. Your cheerfulness and organization are a blessing. I am also grateful for my editor, Jamey

Bennett, for agreeing to review my work, helping me turn my thoughts and typos into something worthwhile.

To all of the doctors, midwives and care providers that practice true integrative medicine, your patients, mothers such as myself, are truly blessed to have access to the absolute best medical care available today. We sincerely thank you.

Finally, to the mothers everywhere that purchase and use my book as a tool, as they aspire to greatness in the noble calling that is motherhood. May your children rise up to call you blessed!

Introduction

My journey into the world of natural health does not resemble the picturesque country lifestyle we all imagine. While my childhood memories are certainly wonderful, they do not include herb walks or bottling herbal extracts. We were quite the modern family, relying heavily on "modern" medicine and for over two years during my high school days I survived on cola, pizza bagels and baked potatoes, complete with a slab of margarine and artificial bacon bits.

Yet, when I became a mother myself, I began to take notice of this new trend towards natural living. I opted for a natural childbirth and was curious as to what other benefits a natural lifestyle might have to offer. This seemingly small decision changed my outlook and my career goals. I began to devour every herb book I could get my hands onto, although there seemed to be a lack of consistent and reliable material at the time, and eventually enrolled in multiple herbal educational programs. Of course, all of this led to my decision to begin an herbal consulting and educating business, Vintage Remedies.

My goals through my business have always centered around sharing what I have learned throughout the years. Every time I discovered something new that had direct benefits for my family, I grew more and more excited and knew I just had to share it with other moms! Through this passion, I have written many books, developed the curriculum for the Vintage Remedies School of Natural Health, which educates families around the globe on the topic of herbal medicine, and am proud to now offer this latest work.

I hope this book becomes a useful, go-to guide in your home, and that is is a blessing to you and your family, whether it is the very first book about natural health that you have read, or your family has already established a thoroughly natural lifestyle.

Jessie Hawkins, MH
wife and mommy

Section One: The Herbal Primer

What is herbalism?

The concept of botanical medicine or herbalism is, as we know, not a new concept at all. Every ancient civilization until recently in history had a strong focus on plant medicine, and offered many experienced professionals to serve as community herbalists. Yet, our modern renewed interest in the topic is often marred with a cloud of confusion, as much of our information comes second hand or from unreliable sources. So, before we can really dig into herbal medicine, it is often beneficial to return to the basic concepts, asking ourselves the simple question, what is herbalism?

Often confused with homeopathy, herbalism is the branch of medicine that combines the art and science of employing plant matter for promoting health and treating illness. While pharmaceuticals are refined single compounds, or more commonly, synthetic versions of refined single compounds, an herb contains hundreds or even thousands of compounds, which work together in a systematic manner to promote wellness in a safe and effective way.

While there is a dramatic difference in the ingredients of a typical herbal remedy and a typical pharmaceutical remedy, the principles behind their uses are very similar. For an inflammatory condition, both systems would use anti-inflammatory treatments. Both forms of medicine combat the illness directly, although herbal medicine is also going to follow a holistic model of care and simultaneously work on boosting our body's own mechanisms, while seeking out any underlying cause for the illness, as opposed to allopathic medicine (the term given to conventional medicine utilizing pharmaceuticals) which simply combats the symptoms and considers the job complete.

Homeopathy, on the other hand, is an entirely different system of medicine. This system is approximately two hundred years old and is based on two Greek words meaning "similar" and "suffering". It operates by three main principles. The first principle is that "like cures like". This means that an inflammatory condition would not be treated with anti-inflammatory remedies, rather inflammatory. This is based on the belief that the body responds to these remedies by increasing its own natural anti-inflammatory response.

Next, we have the concept of "single remedy". This is exactly how it sounds; essentially homeopathy strives to focus on single remedies, as opposed to compounded formulas that are common in other types of medicine. It also results in literally hundreds of possible treatment options, which often require the assistance of a professional homeopath, an individual that is trained to help others choose exactly which remedy is best for them. While many homeopathic therapies can be used effectively at home, these professionals help sift between the many options available, providing the best solution specifically suited to both the individual and the health concern. The final concept is the "minimal dose". Homeopathic remedies are heavily diluted. The stronger medicines are in ratios as high as 1 molecule of the remedy to 1 trillion molecules of water. This heavy dilution leads to a relatively safe system. Using homeopathy is generally considered harmless, since the wrong remedy is not nearly enough to be toxic to the body.

Unfortunately, with the constant confusion between the two natural medicine options, this comfort with safety has been often transferred to botanical medicines and other natural supplements. The rationale of "after all, its natural so it can't harm me" is entirely untrue and unsafe. Herbal medicines and most other supplements are not heavily diluted and do not work in minimal doses. They have measurable effects on the body and these effects can cause harm when used incorrectly.

Other forms of natural medicine include Bach flower remedies and TCM or Traditional Chinese Medicine. Bach flower remedies are based on the work of Dr. Edward Bach, and can actually fall under the homeopathy classification, since they also operate on similar principles. The difference, however, is that flower remedies are basically to treat emotional problems and stresses, and just like the name implies, are made from flowering plants. Traditional Chinese medicine is also often confused with Western herbalism, as it also involves the use of herbal medicine. The two are very similar, in fact, although there are dramatic differences beneath the surface.

TCM is a system of various healing practices that have been used in China for several thousand years. This includes herbal treatments, massage, acupuncture and other practices. It is based on a number of philosophies including the yin yang theory, the five elements, and the human meridian system. It does not operate within the contemporary scientific paradigm, but many physicians have successfully blended the two. Likewise, Ayurveda is the system of healthcare that is native to the Indian subcontinent. It is based on two words meaning "life" and "knowledge" and is widely used among millions of modern individuals. Like TCM, Ayurveda combines philosophical ideas with various healing modalities such as herbalism.

History of Botanical Medicine

Botanical medicine, also called herbalism or phytotherapy, is nearly as old as man. When Adam and Eve left the garden, the world became a place where illness and death were a part of daily life, and hard work defined our days here. Yet, along with that curse came blessings in disguise. With the promise of an eternal remedy also came thorns and thistles. Thistles are most notable to me, as they are not only a burdensome lawn weed, but also a potent rejuvenating plant in botanical medicine.

From the thistle family, we find artichokes, powerful vegetables that are rich in Vitamin C, folate, magnesium, potassium, fiber, iron and protein. They also contain a phytochemical called cynarin, which improves liver function, lowers cholesterol, aids digestion and speeds blood clotting. Not bad for a lowly thistle. From the same family comes milk thistle, which is commonly used throughout the world as a liver tonic. Milk thistle helps to rejuvenate the liver, which is our detoxification organ. When the liver is sluggish, elimination of excess hormones, toxins and other miscellaneous substances is hindered, which can then lead to numerous health concerns. Again, who knew a lawn weed had so many uses!

Actually many individuals and professionals throughout history knew. Though they may not have understood the exact compounds and mechanisms the way that we do today, they certainly knew what effects could be expected through intake of specific herbs and foods.

This plant medicine was the staple of all medical practices from ancient Egypt to the Israelites, through the reign of Rome and even the discovery of a New World. Physicians practiced with advanced therapies combined with ancient surgical techniques, while community herbalists, who were generally well respected individuals such as Martin Luther's wife, Katherine, assisted families with more basic concerns. Mothers knew how to use homemade preparations just like our modern moms know how to browse the aisles of the pharmacy. These skills and practices were documented in old fashioned medical journals and passed down from mother to daughter, herbalist to mentor, and physician to student through apprenticeship and personal instruction.

All of this began to change in the last few hundred years. As additional substances were introduced to the medical field, these historic practices began to be dismissed by the new professionals, and mistrust was spread among the general population. Soon the natural methods became more and more obscure as families discontinued taking responsibility for their own health, preferring to hand the decision making over to the professional physicians with their new therapies, which were not suitable for home preparation. The use of botanical medicine dwindled, although it never did fully exit the scene, and medicine began to change even further with the discovery of the "germ" and then antibiotics.

These substances became the new wonder drugs and few questioned the appropriate use of medicine, instead basking in the newfound discoveries. Of course, these discoveries were quite impressive and have made great strides in the general health of the population, but had the focus remained on natural remedies, these advancements could have had the potential to take us even further today. Overuse of antibiotics has led to antibiotic resistant bacteria, what the World Health Organization has termed one of the most pressing concerns of our day, and an overemphasis on creating sterile environments has led to weakened and even "bored" immune systems, which often turn to attack the body (known as autoimmune disorders), yet are not strong enough to fight off more serious infections. While research exists to show us that antibiotics are not to be taken as frequently as we tend to, and that frequent exposure to milder "germs" keeps the immune system in tip top shape, preventing common childhood disorders such as asthma, our priorities have changed so significantly, that these new truths are generally hard to swallow, let alone understand.

Botanical medicine has never been intended to function as "alternative" medicine, and I have met very few herbalists and wellness professionals that are truly against what we call allopathic medicine, referring to the mainstream or conventional medical practices. Historic use also combines botanicals with other practices, though these changed greatly depending on the culture and their religious beliefs. Ironically enough, these "other practices" are often the ones that give us a good laugh at historic medicine, and modern science has debunked, while the herbal medicines have stood the test of time and rigorous scientific trial. For example, the Egyptians practiced a form of religious medicine, based on beliefs in their specific gods and worldview. These are often mocked, which is understandable, but few can laugh at the impressive ability to mummify a body, preserving it for many years through the use of natural antiseptics and herbal solutions.

Nonetheless, the advancements modern medicine has made are nothing to mock, as antibiotics have saved countless lives. The understanding of pathology has brought about an entirely new era in health, and other medical procedures, especially those found in sports medicine and emergency medicine, are also life savers. No herbalist would dispute that, and most would encourage clients and individuals to seek out these treatments when appropriate.

So, why do we use herbal treatments, if we are not "against" the use of medical treatments? We use them because they are more effective and appropriate for many other medical complications or illnesses. When we face minor viral or bacterial infections, chronic health concerns and even acute medical problems, herbs offer another choice in medicine with fewer side effects (some would argue no side effects), a much better safety track record, and reliable results. Why turn to the "big guns" when we are not facing such dire circumstances?

Herbs offer an intermediate course of action for those times that do not require advanced, usually risky interventions (such as surgery or strong pharmaceuticals), but do require a response for healing. Herbs have stood the test of time, are food-like substances and readily assimilated by the body. Unlike the "new" drugs coming onto the market every couple of months, only to be removed due to dangerous side effects, most herbs have been taken in medicinal amounts for many centuries, if not more. When treating our loved ones and children, this is a safety record that is not to be dismissed.

Worldwide experts also agree, natural medicines are reliable, readily available, more cost effective and most importantly, more effective. Many organizations, including the World Health Organization, have officially recognized the importance of natural medicine, and taken measures to ensure the future availability of these options, as well as the professionals to assist with choosing which option is best.

Another benefit of natural medicine is the ability to place the responsibility of the family's health back into the hands of the family members, where it belongs. Experts all agree that the intuition and oversight of a mother is an invaluable diagnostic tool for assessing the condition of a child, and only the individual can accurately determine what the body is feeling and what lifestyle changes may have contributed to potential health concerns. Placing the burden of responsibility on the physician, who is generally given 10-15 minutes to assess and treat each patient is unrealistic. As a mother, I can vouch for the difference in quality of care my children receive when the family physician and I work together in caring for the health of my children, as opposed to simply bringing in a child with a cough or fever and expecting an accurate diagnosis and simple one-step treatment. The benefits don't end in the feeling of accomplishment I experience as a mother. Our bank account notices a difference, as it is not hit as hard by unnecessary prescriptions and follow-up visits to verify the working diagnosis. Most importantly, my children's health is significantly improved. Each health concern is faced head-on with supplementation of herbs and natural remedies, the diagnostic skills of a physician, determined by physical examination of the child, combined with the significant details provided by an attentive mother, and harsher, more risky interventions are kept at bay, as the last resort, which are rarely found to be necessary.

When we begin to combine the art of natural medicine with the advancements of conventional medicine, we realize that we have some of the best healthcare history has seen.

Prevention

Utilizing natural medicine is much more complex than purchasing a few tinctures at the local health food store and trashing the over the counter remedies already in our medicine chests. Natural medicine is a way of life that can be adapted through a period of time, and passed down to our children and their children. Ignoring the essential lifestyle differences often renders natural medicine ineffective, as the key to health lies in prevention and early intervention, when at all possible. When we neglect these basic concepts, we often find ourselves in a place that requires the "big guns" of drastic intervention to maintain health.

These simple concepts are not difficult to adapt by any means, but are perhaps some of the most misunderstood principles of health. Some take the stance that we are all heading towards death, so why not enjoy life while we have it. To whom I say, how can we enjoy life if we are dealing with unnecessary health problems throughout our days?

Others tell us not to place too much emphasis on the health of our bodies, as they are only temporary, after all, and we do not want to risk setting up a "false idol". Again, I find myself agreeing to disagree, as we can usually all understand the importance of maintaining the health of our bank accounts, raising our children to make wise choices and working hard to provide for our families. Furthermore, would we abandon our common safety measures, since these our only temporary bodies and we don't want to place too much attention on them? I think not. Why would taking care of our bodies not fall under the same classification of responsibility? Especially when research tells us that the majority of our modern health concerns are directly linked to lifestyle and dietary choices?

While the arguments may go on and on, the bottom line is that we cannot expect to experience physical health if we choose to ignore the critical topic of prevention. As the old adage assures us, an ounce of prevention is worth a pound of cure. Quite literally, the absolute best remedy for any physical concern is to focus on prevention, as we never have to concern ourselves with a cure when we avoid the health problem outright.

A healthy lifestyle includes plenty of physical activity. We all know this, but often choose to ignore the real benefits provided by simply adding a bit of physical fitness to the weekly routine. This can be as simple as walking 15-20 minutes each morning to start the day out right, or can be as intense as heading to the gym each afternoon for an hour long rigorous workout.

Regardless of personal preference, exercise and physical activity of any kind is proven to bring about multiple health benefits, including maintaining a healthy body weight, preventing osteoporosis, regulating glucose levels, treating obesity related health problems and so much more. The bottom line: get more exercise into the routine! If that is not enough to be convincing, consider this: exercise also helps to boost daytime energy levels. Feeling sluggish lately? Exercise!

Recent scientific research has shown us the importance of hygienic practices in the avoidance of contagious illness. We have to be careful to use this tool wisely. Striving for a total avoidance of all "germs" can lead to other health problems, so the key is to emphasize hand washing after contact with contagious illness, after bathroom activities, and before consuming or preparing food. On the flip side, we want to be careful not to focus too much on using antibacterial soaps and cleaners. Washing hands with plain soap helps to prevent the spread of disease, and maintaining a clean home with healthy cleaners, which will remove dirt and grime but not attempt to sterilize the area. This offers the best prevention of both modern day chronic concerns and traditional communicable diseases.

The Whole Foods Diet

Another main contributor to prevention involves making adjustments to the diet. Our standard American diet (also known as the SAD) has been directly linked to many health disorders, which are not found in regions that have remained with a traditional whole foods diet.

Throughout this book, and any other book featuring natural remedies, the importance of a whole foods diet is emphasized. Yet, with so many differing and often conflicting opinions about what constitutes a healthy diet (which foods are unhealthy and how we should consume our foods), it is no wonder that the average individual is confused about nutrition.

Considering what a critical role our dietary intake plays in our overall health, during both the prevention and treatment phases, it is important to clarify what history and science tell us about the foods our bodies were designed to consume.

Unfortunately, much of what can be found at the local grocer should not really be considered food. Sure, it is edible, but real food provides nourishment to our bodies, sustaining life and offering vital substances for optimal health. When we drive through a line and pick up a bag at the final window or purchase ready made meals in a box off a shelf, our bellies may stop telling us that they are hungry, but our bodies have not been nourished.

Hippocrates told us to let our food be our medicine. In a world that relied on herbs and other plants for healing as well as culinary staples, this would have been easy to understand. Yet, today we have grocery stores full of edible items that are not real food, pharmacies that are full of manmade substances, many of which are nothing more than synthetic copies of actual plant extracts, and chronic health concerns that research tells us can be prevented, but as a society we have simply accepted as part of the aging process.

Yet, our bodies were not created to live in such a manner. We were created and placed into a world that offers everything we need for health, including nourishing foods and botanical medicines that our bodies readily process and utilize. Plant medicine has sustained the population for millennia, and when combined with our modern scientific understandings about pathogens and hygiene practices, we can have some of the best healthcare that history has ever seen.

Herbs are readily assimilated by our bodies because they are actually food. Basil, for example, is a great adaptogen, helping our bodies overcome stress and environmental changes. Yet, basil is also a delicious seasoning that is added liberally to the diet through pesto and other pasta dishes and as a flavoring agent to numerous other meals. Boosting our intake of fresh, whole foods ensures that our bodies have these benefits in the system daily, and when larger doses are necessary for treatment, instead of prevention, our bodies readily recognize and assimilate these compounds, as they were designed for the intake of these substances.

The whole foods diet refers to the way that we handle and treat the foods as they make their way from the farmer's field to our plates. In an ideal world, these foods would be plucked directly from the organic back yard garden, which is rich in healthy soil, and brought into the kitchen for preparation just prior to consumption. However, this is obviously not possible in every season of the year, and very few individuals still maintain a vegetable garden in their own yards.

So, we adapt by attempting to stick as close to this model as we can in our modern lives. The farther a food goes between the ground to the table, and the more "improvements" we make on it, the fewer benefits it actually offers our bodies. For example, we know that the actual content of vitamins and minerals decreases substantially as a food travels long periods from farmer to table. When we take into consideration assorted processing methods that it might see, these nutrients are decreased even further, so that the actual condition the food arrives to our table in is nothing like real food.

When the food comes fresh from a local farmer or farmer's market, or even a grocer that features local produce, we obviously call the food fresh and local, two terms we are already familiar with. When the food comes intact, without any "improvements" or treatments, such as fortification or processing, we call the food whole. So fresh whole foods would resemble those that were plucked from our backyards in our dream gardens mentioned above.

Real, whole food contains three main macronutrients and dozens of micronutrients. Macronutrients include fats, carbohydrates and proteins. Contrary to common dieting myths, all three of these substances are necessary to healthy living. Fats and carbohydrates are not detriments to the diet, but our modern food choices contain unhealthy versions of these healthy nutrients.

Fats

Fats are necessary for optimal brain functioning, and nearly every system in our body requires fat for energy. Essential fatty acids can help balance inflammation in the body, which is a contributing factor for many modern health concerns.

While many diets focus on a reduction of overall fat intake for reducing bodily fat stores, this is not ideal for weight loss or preventative health. Fat is not the villain society has made it out to be, but certain types of fat can lead to health problems. Moderate intake of healthy fats is not only acceptable in a healthy diet, it is a beneficial part, not to be neglected.

The most common "bad" fat is hydrogenated oil. These oils are not in their natural form; they have been artificially changed, making them saturated. Butter and many tropical oils such as palm and coconut are naturally saturated. This is not a bad thing, in moderation, but the hydrogenated oils are a cause of many health problems and have thus been banned by many European countries and even some US cities.

Hydrogenated oils prevent the body's use of omega 3 and omega 6 fatty acids, causing a decrease in healthy functioning. These fats have been directly linked with increased cholesterol levels, heart disease, decrease in attention span (especially among children), and inflammation in the body, which results in numerous health disorders, as we will see in the next section.

Most animal fats, especially from animals that have been treated with antibiotics and fed non-organic foods are fats to be maintained in moderation. The reason for this is that toxins tend to accumulate in the fat stores of animals. Consuming these fatty foods can lead to consumption of a variety of unhealthy substances. Instead, opt for healthier oil choices based on the intended use of the oil. Generally speaking, fats that will be heated should be saturated, since they are more stable, while fats that will be consumed at room temperature (in a salad dressing for example) should be unsaturated.

Healthy fat choices include nut butters, fish oils, vegetables such as avocado, grains such as flax, and moderate amounts of tropical oils, organic butter and cheese.

Carbohydrates

Carbohydrates are vital to our health, as our bodies literally burn them for energy, just like our cars use fuel. More recently, they have been blamed for our weight problems, but much of this is actually related to the type of carbohydrates that most of us consume, not the consumption of carbohydrates themselves. The resulting "low carb" diets usually leave the dieter with a low fiber intake, high cholesterol, and often a deficiency in many vitamins and minerals, which in turn lead to additional health concerns. Worse yet, long term studies on these diets do not show that they can bring about lasting weight loss. However, a reduction in the poor carbohydrate choices and an increase in healthy carbohydrate choices leads to a healthier body, which usually also means a reduction in excess weight.

Grains are rich in carbohydrates, and throughout history have been revered as the "staff of life", "our daily bread" and other noble titles, suggesting a primary role in the diet. Of course, throughout much of history, bread and grains were not considered synonyms with wheat or flour. Bread was made from a blend of grains, often combined with beans or bean flour. Flour was always whole wheat, unless it was served to the extremely wealthy, and was generally pretty fresh, unlike the white processed powder we purchase at a grocer's.

Other healthy carbohydrate choices include millet, quinoa, rye, lentils, wild rice and, of course, fruits and vegetables. Unhealthy carbohydrates include the "white" foods, white sugar, white flour and any other processed version of the two. These are best avoided altogether, although that can be difficult in real life. In the Hawkins' home, we focus on healthy carbohydrate choices at home so that when we are guests in another, we can politely enjoy whatever is presented to us.

Proteins

Proteins are the building blocks of the body. Pregnant women, growing children and body builders have a need for increased amounts of protein, but the rest of us need much less that the average diet takes in. Part of this is due to the overemphasis popular diets have placed on avoidance of fats and carbohydrates. Like our other macronutrients, protein can come from healthy and unhealthy sources.

Legumes, beans, nuts, and many vegetables and grains offer protein, although our most popular source of protein is animal meat. Generally, whole foods vegetable sources of protein are all healthy choices in moderation. The key is to take in a variety of vegetarian protein choices to prevent deficiencies of certain amino acids. Healthy vegetarian protein sources include brown rice, oats, wheat, broccoli, but animal protein sources can vary greatly as far as nutritional value. Lean meats such as chicken and beef are ideal, while pork, shellfish and other foods listed in Leviticus 11 as "unclean" tend to carry more toxins and disease, according to modern research.

In addition to the processing of foods, many other substances are added to the product before it hits the shelves as well. This can include substances designed to alter the color or flavor of the item, substances that extend the shelf life, allowing the "food" to sit on the shelves longer at both the store and in our pantries, and substances that are literally cheap imitations of more expensive, yet nutritious products. These alterations are a boon to the manufacturer as they prevent spoilage and make the food product taste better with minimal cost. Yet, these enhancements come at a hefty cost to the consumer that falls for the artificially reduced pricing on the shelf.

Artificial colors and flavors have been implicated in numerous trials to cause hyperactivity in children and decrease the attention span. The effects of these substances are so great that many parents have been able to remove ADHD medication from their daily routine by simply altering the diet, omitting these substances. These substances offer no nutritional benefit, and simply exist to enhance the appearance of the food (or often, candy) and mask the lack of actual flavor in a product, so that more expensive, yet flavorful additives (such as real vanilla extract) can be avoided. Whole foods are naturally rich in both color and flavor, with a bright rainbow of fruits and vegetables to choose from, and plenty of their own scent and flavor.

Hydrogenated oils have already been discussed, but will be mentioned again since they are commonly found in so many foods readily available at any corner grocer. Most crackers, including whole wheat crackers, cheese crackers, and pretzels, most candies, many peanut butters, toaster pastries, microwave popcorns and most other snack foods, especially those considered to be "healthy" contain hydrogenated oils. These are foods we often give very young babies and toddlers, and schools readily pass out to children, under the belief that they are a healthy food, because of the low sugar content. Considering that these oils take many weeks to be fully eliminated from our systems, this is an important and lasting change to make in the home.

Likewise, refined or "white" foods are generally understood to be unhealthy, but that seldom stops us from consuming them. Very few foods are naturally white. Sugar and flour are both brown when produced naturally, but are turned white through a refining process. This process also removes any nutrients that were previously found in the food, causing them to create drastic changes in blood sugar, raising them at first, but digesting quickly, causing "crashing" reductions in blood sugar, and rendering them useless as a "health food". Instead, when these items are consumed in their natural state, they are much better for the body as a whole. Sugar can be tolerated, as the minerals necessary for processing are also consumed, and breads can actually be a healthy contribution, instead of something to avoid or keep under moderation.

High fructose corn syrup is an inexpensive and heavily processed form of sugar. Corn is also one of the most genetically modified foods grown today. The exact process of growing fields full of corn and turning it into a sugary syrup is quite complex and quite disturbing. The bottom line is that high fructose corn syrup is not a whole food by any stretch of the imagination. While studies are beginning to come in suggesting that it can lead to obesity, liver damage and many other health concerns, the soda industry is also funding research to attempt to prove it is safe. Quite frankly, I don't need to wait on agreed upon "proof" that the substance is not a healthy choice for my family. Avoiding ingredients that have been so processed that they basically become artificial foods is a basic principle of a whole foods diet.

Quick Checklist of Artificial Ingredients to Avoid

- Hydrogenated oils
- Artificial colors
- Artificial flavors
- Monosodium glutamate (or any of its pseudonyms)
- "White" foods . . . white flour, white sugar, etc.
- Fortified foods
- High fructose corn syrup

Foods likely to contain these ingredients:

- Crackers (wheat crackers, cheddar crackers and even pretzels)
- Most conventional candy products
- Juice "drinks"
- Soup, even organic soup
- Soft drinks
- Boxed cereals
- Butter substitute spreads

Immunity

Our final step in prevention focuses on boosting immunity. Aside from the benefits found in balanced hygienic practices and the boost to our body provided by a healthy whole foods diet, our immune system can be directly affected by immune-boosting or regulating herbal supplements.

These supplements are not always healthy for daily use, but can be added to the routine during times that we know we face increased risk of becoming ill.

For example, our family often travels across the country to visit some relatives. My children are young and we usually take an early morning or late night flight in hopes of allowing them to sleep for a portion of the trip. Yet, the excitement of flying in a plane, anticipation of visiting the beach and an amusement park, and the eagerness to see family members that have been missed often leads to a restless flight. The temptation is to keep them occupied with small treats along the way for good behavior. But we know that if we consistently fill their little bodies with small amounts of sugar, while they are excited and exposed to pathogens from a different region of the country than their bodies are accustomed to, we can go right ahead and plan on staying home for a large part of the trip to battle whatever illness made its way into their bodies.

We choose instead, to take along our own healthy treats to keep their tummies filled and minds occupied. We reduce exposure to sugar, which can lower the immune response by forty percent for up to four hours. Even natural sugars or small amounts of sugar can lead to this reduction. Next, we ensure that their bodies have had enough sleep, to avoid the decreased immune response that is caused by stress or overexcitement. Finally, we supplement their systems with herbal assistance for the days before and after such a trip.

Another situation that generally causes us to exercise an increased vigilance towards immunity includes the back-to-school week in early fall, shortly after when our friends all begin taking their flu vaccines, and we know the official flu season has begun, and during the winter holidays when we are exposed to many different visitors in a short time period. Birthday parties, festivals, and any time we see an increase in excitement or exposure to illness also usually causes us to begin short term supplementation with immune boosting herbs.

One of the most common herbs for immune function is a Chinese legume names astragalus. This herb is known to boost the white blood cell count, those "fighter" cells that are responsible for fighting off pathogens. I like the Herbs for Kids brand plain astragalus glycerite. It is mild and gentle, and my children do not even notice the taste when I drop their dose into a glass of water. For us adults, I buy an adult glycerite, as I prefer the mild flavor that glycerin extracts offer.

Another herb widely used for immunity is elderberry. This berry offers great immune stimulating properties and the taste is similar to that of blueberry pancake syrup, only thicker and without the sugary taste. For early treatment of common viral illnesses, the syrup can be purchased with a blend of herbs in the formula. Echinacea is the most common addition, but other cough and cold related herbs can be found. Considering the vast options, it is crucial to double check the ingredient list to ensure that the right blend is purchased for prevention or treatment.

Garlic is an herb that is also a delicious food, and can be liberally added to the diet. This herb boosts immunity, and when I know I have been exposed to something, I like to make homemade garlic bread with lots and lots of fresh, yummy garlic to boost my immune system. For those that do not like the taste of garlic, an odorless capsule is available for similar benefits. Garlic can have mild blood thinning effects, so those scheduled for a surgical procedure should discontinue use 5-7 days prior to the procedure, and those on, or avoiding, blood thinners should check with the family physician or wholistic consultant for potential interactions.

In addition to our herbal and dietary methods of prevention, a couple of small lifestyle changes can lead to healthier bodies as well. Choosing to set aside one day a week for a break from the daily stress and busyness not only brings about a calm and relaxed state of mind, it allows the entire body to rest, which means that the immune system is better suited to fight off illness. Relaxing around the table during mealtime also helps to ensure that our food is properly digested and nutrients are absorbed, reducing nutrient deficiencies, and again effecting the overall health of the body in a positive way.

Tips to Boost Immunity During Increased Exposure:

Avoid sugars if at all possible
Cleanse hands with an essential oil spray or soap and water
Bring clean water for maintaining hydration
Pack healthy snacks
Supplement with astragalus, elderberry or garlic

Creating New Family Ways

As we begin to make these changes in our lifestyles, our children begin to notice the differences and begin to adapt them to their lives. Instead of learning how to buy the foods that have been marked down to be inexpensive, they learn how to stretch their grocery dollars by purchasing whole food ingredients and baking their own goods.

Which brings up another point, how many of us became adults fully prepared to cook healthy meals for a family? Then when we add in the necessary budget restraints, and a problem is compounded. Yet, these new habits of the home will be picked up by the younger members of our families, and adapted to their own lifestyles, impacting the health of our grandchildren and their children, as these new family ways take root.

Cooking whole food meals from healthy and fresh ingredients teaches our children the importance of prevention and nutrition, instead of allowing them to grow up believing that breakfast comes from a box and brownies come from a paper bag on the shelf.

Another habit to pass along is the inclusion of a farmer's market or CSA (community supported agriculture) into the lifestyle. This provides multiple benefits. Not only do we have the opportunity to purchase fresh, often organic produce and meats directly from the farmer, cutting out the middleman means a better price value for us, and more profit for the small farmer for their hard work. Everyone benefits, including our children, who grow up with the knowledge of where the food comes from (no, milk does not come from the grocery store) and cherish the memories of playing outside with friends while waiting for their weekly share, or chatting with the farmers that actually grew and harvested much of their food. These children are much more likely to value local and healthy food as adults than those that were only given the stale vegetables on the grocer's shelf that were plucked weeks ago and traveled thousands of miles to our homes.

Likewise, when we are not quick to turn to over the counter remedies or head to the family physician requesting an antibiotic long before we know what illness we are even dealing with, instead choosing to alter the diet and schedule for the day, supplementing with immune boosting herbs and treating with gentle, natural remedies, our children learn how to properly use these medications and can avoid the learning curves we faced to provide these benefits for our families. While we all readily know how to use ibuprofen and acetaminophen, few of us were raised with a working knowledge of when and how to use wild cherry bark or goldenseal root. Passing this knowledge on to our children again provides benefits that can then impact generation after generation for the better. Considering the lifelong problems and benefits caused by the nutritional and environmental decisions made in pregnancy, these small lifestyle habits could literally make a great difference.

For families that have already begun with less than ideal habits, this does not have to be a daunting task. True and lasting changes to the diet and health habits are only made one way: slowly. Altering the diet overnight not only leads to rejection from little taste buds that have grown accustomed to the nutrition lacking items in the grocery shelves, it leads to frustration, and strong detoxification in the body as the body is literally shocked with these major changes. This can result in diarrhea, cold like symptoms and general fatigue, none of which encourage an individual to "keep it up".

Some easy ways to begin change include blending whole wheat flour into a favorite cookie recipe. Begin with something small, maybe 10% or even 15%. Gradually increase the amount by about 5% each time, and before long, the whole family has adapted to whole wheat cookies. Once that step is down, work on changing to a whole foods sugar, instead of white sugar. We do this the same way we changed the type of flour, and eventually we have a healthy cookie that we can feel good about providing to the family.

Integrative Medicine

There are many terms to define the combination of both natural methods with our modern allopathic options. This can be referred to as blended medicine, integrated medicine, inclusive medicine, and so on. Regardless of the preferred term, the concept is the same: focus on natural treatments, gradually working our way to the more dangerous and aggressive treatments, stopping when the desired results have been achieved.

Many care providers have already begun to undertake this concept on their own, including herbal and dietary remedies into their daily practice of medicine. Some physicians refer out to trained nutritionists and herbalists, while others have gone as far as to actually enroll in educational courses to learn more about these treatment options so that they can personally blend the two successfully. When this happens, we generally refer to the professional as a physician practicing wholistic (often spelled holistic) medicine, meaning that he or she focuses on the whole body and person, not only the problematic part.

During medical school, in a very few locations, a physician can actually choose to learn about natural medicine right alongside allopathic medicine, learning from the start how to incorporate and successfully blend the two approaches for optimal care. These physicians do not earn the title of M.D. or medical doctor, rather they are known as N.D.s or naturopathic doctors. Naturopathic doctors are licensed to practice medicine in many states, and can offer the same allopathic benefits that an M.D. can offer, with the added benefit of experience in holistic health. These care providers are usually exceptional.

Another type of professional, however, also carries the name of N.D. Traditional or classical naturopathic doctors are not doctors as we have learned to use the term, rather they are classical doctors, choosing to use the earliest meaning of the word "teacher". These are unlicensed professionals, much like an herbalist or homeopath, and are trained specifically in natural health. While they do not carry a license to practice allopathic medicine, and are not trained in allopathic medicine, they do have quite a bit to offer in terms of a vast area of experience within the natural medicinal realm. I personally find it unfortunate that the two share a name, as it has brought about quite a bit of tension among the professionals, and quite a bit of confusion among patients or clients. When seeking out a holistic care provider, it is important to fully understand exactly what the provider is trained and licensed by the state to do for his or her patients, to ensure that the right provider is chosen for the right job.

When a health situation arises in a home that chooses to utilize natural remedies and integrative medicine, the basic actions taken regardless of the type of health care professional that assists. We begin with the least invasive treatment, and move step by step through our options, only moving forward as the situation requires, saving the bigger moves such as surgical procedures for extreme situations.

Many times, we will find that a situation can be effectively treated with little more than lifestyle changes and nutritional support. Some larger situations may require botanical remedies or even pharmaceuticals, and our crisis situations are treated with the serious, last resort treatments.

When we follow this outline, there is no reason to worry about needless interventions, invasive procedures or overuse of pharmaceuticals. We have begun with the safest, most gentle treatment, and only moved to the latter steps if necessary.

Step One: Focus on Lifestyle and Dietary Decisions

This step simply involves ensuring adequate rest in the day, ensuring plenty of time for the body to work on its own defenses, allowing the immune system to heal itself. Reducing the stressful activities in the day, as much as is possible and relaxing about routine activities all reduce the potential for the body to inhibit its own natural function.

During this time, we also pay close attention to the diet, reducing sugar and other items that can hinder our immune function, and focusing on healthy whole foods to ensure the body has everything it needs to work on preventing illness.

Step Two: Immune Support

When that is not enough, we focus our attention on assisting the immune function with supportive herbs and a class of herbs called adaptogens. These herbs are a step further from the dietary changes, but still extremely safe and effective. We are not yet looking at treating the actual illness, at this point we are still helping the body work the way it was designed to. The immune boosting herbs we discussed earlier, including astragalus, elderberry extract and when appropriate, garlic are ideal uses for this step.

Adaptogens also help the body face stress and lifestyle changes successfully. Astragalus is an effective adaptogen, as is holy basil and gingko.

Step Three: Botanical Remedies

Sometimes boosting the immune system is still not enough and we need to directly address the problem. When this happens, we begin with botanical or herbal medicines to combat the illness. This step includes all other classifications of herbal medicine, including antibacterial herbs such as goldenseal or Oregon grape root, antifungal herbs such as myrrh or garlic, expectorants, anti-inflammatories, and the many other treatments that come from plants.

Step Four: Pharmaceuticals

This step includes the use of prescription remedies. This is appropriate in situations that might require a more immediate effect than botanical medications usually provide, or for stronger more dangerous illness that requires a more serious action. Antibiotics fall in this heading, as do many strong, yet mildly toxic, over the counter remedies.

Step Five: Physically Invade

This step includes drastic measures such as surgical procedures and high potency pharmaceuticals such as chemotherapy. It is a last resort, when all other steps have failed us, but can still be used in conjunction with other steps along the way. For example, after a surgical procedure, botanical remedies can be taken to speed healing and reduce pain and inflammation from the surgical site, a whole foods diet can play a role in improved energy levels after such procedures and nutrition, lifestyle and immune support can all be key players in preventing a re-occurrence of the situation.

Herbal Medicine Chest

To accomplish all of these things in the home, the average medicine chest is in need of a drastic makeover. In many homes, this is a gradual step, as more and more pharmaceutical remedies are replaced with botanical extracts, and before long, the medicine chest looks less like an aisle in the pharmacy and more like a kitchen pantry or garden preservation project!

While a sudden change in routine can lead to costly purchases and a stash of remedies that might be unfamiliar in both taste and appropriate use to the members of the family, the gradual adjustment avoids these pitfalls, so that path always receives my hearty recommendation.

However, there is certainly something to be said for stocking a well prepared herbal medicine chest. Considering the inconvenience these remedies can cause in the midst of a family illness, when most remedies can only be found at a health food store, knowing that these remedies are readily available in my kitchen certainly makes a mommy sleep better at night.

While the best medicine chest will vary from family to family, to fit each individual's unique needs, there are some basics that are useful to any family, especially when children are in the home. In the Hawkins' home, we make sure our stash always contains the items listed below, although the brand may change slightly according to what is available when I stock up, the purpose and main use will remain the same.

Household Items

- Medicine dropper (for dosing children that are not yet old enough to readily take syrups and other remedies from a spoon)
- Humidifier
- Reliable measuring spoons (quarter, half and whole teaspoon)
- Raw honey (or brown rice syrup for infants)
- Unbleached muslin for compresses
- First aid supplies: bandages, tweezers, cotton swabs, gauze, adhesive tape and hydrogen peroxide

Tinctures or Glycerites

- Astragalus
- Echinacea / Oregon grape root blend
- Garlic Oil
- Herbs for Kids' Garlic Willow oil
- Milk thistle
- Children's composition plus or Herbs for Kids' Temp Assure
- Bilberry
- Gingko
- Holy basil
- Digestive formula including peppermint, ginger, chamomile and fennel
- Herbs for Kids' cherry bark blend (for one child that is prone to respiratory infections)

Other Remedies

- Elderberry syrup
- Elderberry syrup with Echinacea
- Natural Factors' Anti-V formula
- Probiotic blend (one for children, one for adults, both Udo's Choice)
- Kyolic garlic capsules
- Thayer's slippery elm bark tablets
- Witch hazel extract

- Epsom salts
- Nettle capsules
- Nordic Naturals fish oils for children and adults
- New Chapter Organics One Daily multivitamins
- Nordic Naturals Nordic Berries (children's multis)
- Calendula salve
- Arnica ointment
- Owie Balm™ (personal formula)

Dried Herbs

- Chamomile
- Calendula
- Comfrey
- Plantain
- Eucalyptus
- Slippery elm bark
- Blackberry leaf

Essential Oils

- Lavender
- Eucalyptus
- Tea tree
- Lemon
- Peppermint
- Myrrh
- Sweet orange
- Cinnamon

Herbal Safety

According to recent polls, up to 80% of Americans have used natural medicine at some point recently. Modern research tells us that herbs are a reliable and safe way to treat many different ailments. However, before these effective remedies can begin to make their ways back into our homes successfully, a better awareness about herbal safety is in order.

If we can trust these herbs to alter our bodies and cure our disease, we have to acknowledge that these same herbs can do harm when used inappropriately. The most important part of my job as an herbalist, especially when consulting with individual clients, is to stress the use of safety and common sense when self treating with herbs.

This section is certainly not meant to deter the safe use of herbal remedies, but it is written to serve as a reminder that we should always be cautious with any substance we put into the mouths or on the bodies of our family members as we attempt to treat their illnesses. Whether the substance came from a corner drug store, a pharmacist by request of a physician's prescription, or the health food store in a capsule or tincture bottle, we have to remember that safety considerations should always remain on the front of our minds. After all, an overdose is possible with any substance (even water) and drug interactions should always be ruled out prior to dosing.

With that in mind, here are some important safety tips, adapted from a handout designed for use in my consulting practice, that are important to keep in mind before treating any member of your family with home remedies.

Obtain a Diagnosis

Self-diagnosis is, unfortunately, very common among those that utilize natural medicine. In my profession, I often speak with mothers that have not even chosen a family physician and whose children have never been evaluated by a doctor. I have had clients that self diagnosis countless illnesses, including one that diagnosed himself with hypertension based on how he felt, and had never even taken his own blood pressure! This is a practice that I cannot, in good conscience encourage. The ability to diagnose assorted health concerns is an entirely different skill than the ability to choose natural medicines. Even as an experienced herbalist with a busy consulting practice, my children visit our family physician anytime I need a formal diagnosis or additional clarity that helps me choose the right remedy for the concern. Without valuable information that can only be obtained through bloodwork, labwork and a skilled, experienced practitioner, I am forced to rely on my best guess, and if the supposed diagnosis is wrong, then my treatments will likely be wrong as well.

Have a Good Network of Professionals

In addition to the help of a family physician, it is important to have a well trained herbalist or other holistic professional as a resource for wellness information when the situation may develop into something greater than expected. These professionals are trained in the specifics of botanical medicines and can help connect the dots between the medical realm and the natural realm. Graduates of the Vintage Remedies School of Natural Health's herbal education programs are excellent examples of such professionals.

Use Extreme Caution in Young Children

It is never a good idea to medicate any child under the age of 3 (three) unless there is a good understanding of the herbal remedy and a clear diagnosis. Additionally, as with any medication, the correct dosage must be strictly adhered to. Too often we think, "If a little is good, a lot must be better." With medications, this is never the case. We can always add more to the child; it is not so easy to remove it.

Children that are still nursing can "take" herbal medications through the mother's milk, and this is often the best choice.

Finally, if there are any questions or concerns, avoid medicating a young child. Find a holistic professional in the area and discuss the concerns with them. If there are no professionals in the area, many are willing to take out of town clients, offering helpful information via phone or email.

Follow Correct Dosing Guidelines

The manufacturer of the herbal supplement is the best source for dosing information. Many children's herbals are now including helpful weight and age appropriate dosing information on the label. When using an adult herbal for a child (first be sure it is a herb appropriate for a child) or when using a supplement that does not specify exact dosing, keep in mind that the typical dose given is for a 150 pound adult. This means that if you are a 100 pound female, the correct dose is 2/3 of the suggested amount. If you are a 300 pound adult, you will need approximately twice the amount specified.

For some situations, this means that we are literally counting drops of a tincture for a child, so we need to consider that 1 teaspoon is roughly 100 drops (give or take a few depending on the size of your drops!) and 3 teaspoons is a tablespoon.

Use Caution With the Elderly

As we age, our bodies react differently to herbs, and we will require decreasing dosages to achieve the same effect. As a general rule, adults ages 60 and up will require 70% of the typical adult dose, while ages 70 and up will require 60% of the typical adult dosage. Adults over the age of 80 will only need about half of a dose. This is in addition to adjusting for weight.

Here is an example of that in action: Let's use astragalus as our example. This particular package says to take 1 teaspoon, 3 times a day. An 84 year old woman weighing 200 pounds would first determine that her weight calls for 1 and 1/3 teaspoons of the herb. Next she would see that her age calls for only half. Thus her dosage would be 2/3 teaspoon.

Know the Medicine

Before ingesting any herb, we should always know exactly what to expect. This is not just talking to friends of family members, it includes looking at the scientific studies on the herb and making sure we are comfortable with the typical results. When pharmaceuticals are also in the picture, it also includes discussing the medications with our primary care provider.

Purchase Remedies From Reliable Sources

Herbal remedies should only be purchased from a reputable source. Herbs in the US are regulated as supplements, not drugs. This can mean that the potency can vary from brand to brand. Many larger, established companies have labs to test their products and ensure a consistent product. Others go as far as to standardize certain elements within the supplement.

In addition, smaller companies have been caught adulterating their herbals with cheaper imitations. It is always vital to know the source, their standards and their reputation.

Observe for Reactions

Each person is an individual. This means that 99.9% of us can have a certain reaction to something, and that one rare person has a different reaction. This is something known as an idiopathic reaction; idiopathic literally means, "for unknown reasons". Obviously, these are rare, but they do happen. We should always be alert when taking a new herb or food and stay aware of any allergic or adverse reactions. If something unusual happens, the remedy should be discontinued until we locate the source of the occurrence.

Caution in Pregnancy

With few exceptions, women who are pregnant or nursing should not take medicinal amounts of any herb without a thorough working knowledge of herbal medicine or access to an experienced herbalist or care provider with experience in herbal medicine. (Many midwives are also trained in botanical medicine for pregnancy.)

Our placenta serves as a sieve, not a filter, and everything we take will go to the baby. Also, a typical assumption is that an herb that is safe for children is safe for pregnant women. This is not exactly true. This thinking is based on taking smaller amounts of a medication in the hopes that some results will be achieved while serving minimal exposure to the baby. However, certain actions are not justified in the case of pregnancy. The cautions pregnant women observe and the cautions children observe are different since both their bodies and their bodies' needs are different.

If an illness occurs during a pregnancy that requires treatment, botanical medications can still offer a safer and reliable option for the mommy and baby duo, but the exact remedy and dose will need to be determined through consulting with the midwife or physician and other members of the medical birthing team. It is not advisable to treat illness at home without first consulting with a professional with sufficient herbal training.

Appendix Two in the back of this book contains a list of commonly used herbs that should be avoided during pregnancy or lactation.

Avoid Trendy Medicine

Caution should always be used when starting any new health trend. Herbs and health foods go through trends, as do diets. While many of these products actually can be beneficial, many are not, and most are not in the amount typically seen in the fads. Health crazes are just that. Common sense and balance is always the best and healthiest approach.

Obtain Help When Needed

Any self treated illness should be evaluated by a professional if no improvement has been seen after 3-5 days, depending on the severity of the problem. Sometimes, what we are dealing with has changed, as in the case of a virus that brought on a bacterial infection, and our treatment needs to change. Other times, we may be right on track and need nothing to change. Still others, we may have missed a crucial symptom that changes what our treatment should be and the outside eyes will catch that.

Communicate Well

Finally, and most importantly, communication with the care provider is crucial. Typically, during the question portion of the visit (usually with a nurse) they will ask if the patient is taking anything. This is especially important if facing surgery or other major procedures, as certain herbs can change basic things like how the blood clots.

While it is estimated that 80% of Americans take natural supplements, only 25% of that 80% admit to informing their care provider of what they are doing. Not only is this irresponsible, it can be dangerous. If the care provider is hostile to the patient's choices, it is probably time for a change, but an open and honest relationship with a licensed care provider is crucial.

While treating illness at home might seem like a daunting task, the truth is that we regularly administer medications at home with little thought. Ibuprofen, acetaminophen, antihistamines and other similar remedies are mainstays in most homes, and we rarely consult with a professional before dosing up our family members for a little cough or sniffle. From childhood we are trained in the common use of these remedies, yet very few individuals actually have a working knowledge of the actions and side effects of such remedies. With a little experience, these safety measures, and some common sense, herbal remedies can become reliable alternatives and provide safe and effective results.

Pediatric Considerations

When treating children, it is important to remember that not only are their bodies smaller than ours, their bodily systems are usually operating quite differently that ours are. Little tummies are much more permeable than our adult tummies and little bodies typically require much less medicine than the adult equivalent of the same extract.

While we generally divide an adult supplement by the weight of the child to determine the dose, we should also always begin with the mildest dose, only working our way up if necessary. Most extracts offer a range as the correct dose, so the lower number on that range is the staring point. Additionally, many herbalists, including myself, prefer to treat using half doses, twice as often. While this may seem like a pain to remember how much to give every 2 hours, it is a much better treatment protocol for younger children, generally leads to faster recovery, and reduces the actual amount of herb in the body in case of a reaction.

To follow that treatment plan, let's consider an example. We have an echinacea glycerite with a recommended dose of 30-50 drops on the label and are treating our 50 pound 6 year old. The lowest number in the dose range is 30, so we begin there. The child is 1/3 of 150 pounds, so we divide the 30 drops by 3 as well. We are left with a dose of 10 drops. Instead of giving these 10 drops 3 times a day, we opt to administer 5 drops every 2 hours or 4 times a day. If we need to increase the dosage, we can increase it to 6 or even 7 drops. As an added bonus, it is very easy to drop 5-7 drops of an extract into a small cup of juice or even water, making is far less daunting to give a child herbs 5-6 times a day!

Section Two:
The Family Clinic

Acne

What is it? Acne is a common nuisance among teenagers, but the skin problem can plague individuals of all ages. The most common type, acne vulgaris, produces blackheads, whiteheads, and inflammation. The troublesome cysts are caused by acne conglobata. Acne generally presents itself as minor skin eruptions, which typically occur on the face, but can be found all over the body. These blemishes seldom last longer than a week or two, but can come in droves and recurring spots are not exactly considered desirable.

Prevention: Acne can be prevented or at least lessened by ensuring the skin has plenty of exposure to fresh air. Our cosmetic facial covering is notorious for clogging pores and trapping dirt. Natural cosmetics are available, and it is always a good idea to allow the face a few cosmetic free days every so often. A healthy, whole foods diet is another great prevention method, as it ensures that the body has plenty of nutrients and is not attempting to rid itself of numerous toxins that have been introduced through the diet.

Many individuals with acne have the mistaken belief that it is caused by dirty skin, so they attempt to fix this by frequently washing, and even scrubbing the face in an attempt to eliminate the problem. This can actually worsen the problem, as it strips the skin from valuable protective oils, stimulating the production of additional oil. In general, washing the face in the morning and before bedtime is sufficient to maintain clean skin.

Likewise, many with acne also believe, thanks to years of misinformation, that oil based products will worsen the situation and use soaps and cosmetics designed to remove oil from the skin. This also disturbs that careful balance of oil production by the body. Oil actually dissolves oil, so an oil based cleanser can actually dissolve the excess oil on the face, and as it is rinsed away, takes the excess oil with it. This gentle method does not strip the skin, stimulating the production of additional oil, so it is highly effective at balancing the moisturizing properties on the skin.

Treatments: Facial steams have been beneficial to many that suffer from acne. To enjoy a home facial treatment that can also help with facial acne, try the formula below.

Calming Berry Steam

Blend together 2T of each: dried lavender buds, dried chamomile petals, and dried blackberry leaves. Store in a glass jar. To use: scoop out 1T of the blend into a muslin drawstring bag. Place in the sink, under the spout and turn on warm / hot water. Fill the basin about halfway, then turn off the water. Place your (clean, freshly washed) face 6-8 inches above the water line so that the steam can reach you but does not run the risk of burning. Drape a towel over your head to trap the steam. Be careful not to burn your face, as the steam may be very hot! After 5-10 minutes, or when the treatment ceases to be enjoyable, remove the towel and rinse the face with cool water. This steam treatment offers both astringent and anti-inflammatory properties, which are very valuable when acne is present.

Since many tests reveal that those with acne often have higher levels of testosterone and / or androgen in the body, supplementation to adjust this balance is often useful. Milk thistle is a liver supporting herb that helps the body to process and eliminate excess hormones efficiently. Look for a supplement that is standardized to contain 80% silymarin. (Silymarin is the active compound in the plant.)

As a topical treatment, tea tree oil has been shown to be as effective as benzoyl peroxide, but with far fewer side effects. Tea tree oil cannot be applied directly to the skin, as it can easily irritate sensitive tissues, but a solution with up to 25% or even 50% can be effectively used as a spot treatment.

Anti-acne Home Facial

Fruit acids help to eliminate excessive amounts of the protein keratin. They also remove dead skin cells that may clog pores if allowed to remain. To take advantage of these properties, mash a handful of strawberries then apply to the face and neck. Allow to sit for 5-10 minutes before gently removing with a warm, damp cloth. Follow up with the anti-inflammatory actions of chamomile by blotting a strongly brewed tea directly onto the face with a cotton ball.

ADHD

What is it? ADHD (attention-deficit hyperactivity disorder) is one of our modern childhood epidemics. First described by Dr. Heinrich Hoffman in 1845, ADHD is characterized by inattention, hyperactivity and impulsive behavior, but the exact appearance of these symptoms will look differently in every child. The Center for Disease Control estimates that 1 in 13 children have ADHD.

Prevention: Many environmental triggers are known to exacerbate ADHD, or even serve as the tipping point, triggering the onset of the disorder. These include heavy metals, food sensitivities or allergies, nutritional deficiencies, thyroid disorders, and even risky pregnancy interventions. Parenting in a natural, wholistic living manner helps to ensure that these triggers are kept at a minimal level in the developing child's body.

Treatments: One of the most popular and effective treatments for ADHD is to adjust the diet, removing foods that are known to hinder concentration and optimal brain functioning. The most common of these are: hydrogenated oils, artificial colors / flavors, MSG (and its other aliases including autolyzed yeast, hydrolyzed vegetable protein, yeast extract and glutamic acid), preservatives, and most refined or "white" foods, including flours and sugars.

Fish oil supplementation has also proven useful for increasing concentration and enhancing learning in the classroom for students with ADHD. My favorite brand is Nordic Naturals children's DHA.

Many other children have benefited from food sensitivity testing, screening for heavy metals, detoxification, and the gluten free / casein free diet, combined with probiotics and digestive enzymes. The Vintage Remedies website is a great source for tips and recipes for these special diets.

Additionally, certain essential oils have shown to help increase concentration and enhance memory. A blend of lemon, lavender and thyme essential oil lightly diffused throughout the homeschool room or classroom helps to increase concentration, improve memory and promote mental clarity. This provides great benefit in school performance, which is often hindered due to the fact that the unique learning styles of children with ADHD do not often blend with typical classroom styles of teaching.

Alcoholism

What is it? Alcoholism is the dependence on alcohol, accompanied by cravings, a loss of control, withdrawal symptoms and an increased tolerance for the substance. It is usually chronic, lasting a person's entire lifetime and relapses can only be prevented by a lifelong avoidance of the substance. Many individuals use the term alcoholism to describe an enjoyment of alcoholic beverages that may be temporarily overly indulgent, but not an actual dependence on the substance. While that might be a legitimate cause for concern, it is not an example of actual alcoholism.

Prevention: The best way to prevent alcoholism is to avoid alcoholic drinks or drink only in moderation at all times. The consumption of alcohol is an intensely debated topic among American Christians, but other cultures do not experience this stigma, and the consumption of alcohol is more commonplace. Regardless of personal doctrinal beliefs, a healthy lifestyle limits alcohol consumption to "moderate" use, which is defined as 1 drink per day for a female and 1-2 drinks per day for a male.

Treatments: Research has shown that supplementation with kudzu root has been shown to decrease the number of alcoholic drinks a heavy drinker consumes in a day.

Alcoholics often have a thiamin (B1) deficiency and low magnesium levels. This can lead to problems during withdrawal. There is also a direct link between the amount of Vitamin C in the body and the speed of alcohol elimination from the body. A good whole foods multivitamin will provide additional stores of both vitamins, but magnesium is often found as a separate calcium / magnesium blend.

Since alcohol can take a toll on the liver, those that abuse the substance generally have sluggish livers. This can be treated with milk thistle supplementation. Milk thistle has been shown in some trials to even stimulate the regeneration of liver cells, leading to complete recovery. Look for a supplement that is standardized to contain at least 80% silymarin, which is the active compound in the herb.

Finally, a diet rich in antioxidants can help reverse any damage that has happened due to the sluggish liver or excessive alcohol intake.

Allergies

(for seasonal allergies, see hay fever)

What is it? An allergy is an immune response to a food that is mistakenly considered to be harmful by the body. Our immune system has a wonderful memory, creating antibodies against substances it deems harmful, so when this harmless food is ingested again, a series of events are triggered. This includes the production of histamine, a tingling sensation in the mouth, swelling of the tongue and throat, hives, difficulty breathing, vomiting, diarrhea, decrease in blood pressure, and / or stomach cramping, within a matter of minutes after consumption. Serious reactions can lead to loss of consciousness and even death.

Food allergies have become more common in recent years, but no cause or cure has been determined. Emerging science is beginning to consider a link between allergies and our other modern childhood epidemics, such as ADHD, asthma and autism, which is especially interesting when we consider that children facing one of these conditions are more likely to face others as well.

Prevention: Infants are born with immature digestive systems that were specifically designed to digest human milk. The addition of cow milk or other foods to the diet can often be too difficult for the immature system to handle properly, and this can actually lead to increased risk of developing a food allergy, even if there is not a history of allergies in the family.

To combat this risk, infants should not take in any food or drink other than breastmilk (or formula when absolutely necessary) for the first six months of life. Once foods are introduced, gentle, non allergenic choices such as brown rice cereal, many fruits and most vegetables are well suited to offer the child a safe introduction to solid food. Common allergens such as wheat (or any gluten containing grain), nuts, berries, citrus foods, soy, fish and cow milk should be avoided until 24 months of age, when the digestive tract is mature enough to handle them properly. These foods account for 90% of all food allergies. While this does not ensure the child will not develop an allergy, it greatly reduces the risk of aggravating or triggering one.

Treatments: True food allergies should be considered medical emergencies and are treated by standard allopathic care. Natural medicine is aimed at preventing allergies and reducing the symptoms, but a reaction should be treated by a licensed medical professional, given the potentially serious effects it can cause.

While allergies cannot be cured in children or adults, there is evidence that the sensitivity to the food can be lessened, which could potentially save many lives. Allergies range in severity to those that are triggered by ingestion of the food to those that are triggered by simply touching the food to those that are so sensitive that they are triggered by simply being in a room that also contains the food.

In his book, *Healing the New Childhood Epidemics,* Dr. Kenneth Bock discusses methods that DAN! (Defeat Autism Now!) doctors can use to help with this naturally through diet, detoxification and supplementation. Each individual is different, and the protocol is dependent on the allergy and medical history, so we will not cover them here, but there are some common treatments that include: supplementation with fish oils, antifungal medication, probiotic supplementation, extreme restriction of commonly reactive foods, environmental controls (reduced exposure to environmental toxins) and immune system regulators.

Anemia

What is it? Anemia is the term for a situation in which an individual has a red blood cell count that is lower than normal. Red blood cells are the cells that carry oxygen throughout the body, so one of the most common symptoms of anemia is fatigue.

Anemia often affects women, especially during the childbearing years, and children, especially during the later half of the first year of life. The part of the red blood cell that carries the oxygen throughout the body is called hemoglobin, so anemia is often diagnosed by checking the hemoglobin levels in the body, but for a complete diagnosis, a CBC (complete blood count) is often taken. While there are many types of anemias, the most common is iron deficiency anemia.

According to the World Health Organization, up to 80% of the world's population has an iron deficiency, which makes it the most widespread deficiency in the world. Prompt treatment is best, since untreated anemia can lead to developmental delays in children, as well as extreme fatigue and heart problems.

Prevention: Anemia is often difficult to prevent, but iron deficiency can be prevented by ensuring plenty of iron intake through a well balanced and varied diet. Foods rich in Vitamins C and B complex enhance iron absorption, so they are also important in preventing anemia. Foods rich in iron include spinach, animal meats (especially red meats), dark leafy vegetables and organic molasses. One great way to boost iron stores is to pair these foods with those rich in Vitamins C and B complex, such as a spinach salad with strawberries. It is also important to note that milk and calcium in general inhibit iron absorption.

Treatments: Before treating anemia, it is important to obtain a firm diagnosis. Iron supplementation should be taken only when a true deficiency exists, so it should not be added to the daily routine unless a licensed care provider has provided a valid diagnosis.

My personal favorite remedy for anemia is a product called Flora-dix or Flora-vital. Both blends are produced by the Flora Health company. This product is a whole foods supplement, which is easier for the body to absorb. While the increased absorption rates may seem a bit high, the blend does not promote the storage of excessive iron in the body and is even non constipating! It is safe enough for young children (in adjusted doses under constant supervision) and is highly effective. This supplement is a must-have in my home during a pregnancy.

Yellow dock and nettle are two herbs that are naturally rich in iron and can serve as a whole foods supplement. These herbs can be found in tincture or glycerite form at a health food store and taken according the manufacturers directions.

Chlorophyll, the extract known as the "blood of plants", has been used to obtain a quick rise in hemoglobin. Chlorophyll is available in both capsules and liquid form. The liquid often has a minty flavor to it. General dose is 1 teaspoon, twice a day.

Supplementation with vitamin C and B complex helps increase the absorption of iron, and when combined with iron rich foods are a beneficial habit to complement any anemia treatment.

Anxiety

What is it? Anxiety is the term given to a concern, fear, dread or state of nervousness that can be either persistent or directly linked to an upcoming event. While many like to pretend anxiety is nothing more than excessive worrying, the intense apprehension is actually much more than a bad habit for the individual that suffers from anxiety. Anxiety has real, physical symptoms and often leads to "panic attacks". It is important to distinguish between normal anxiety and an anxiety disorder, which is the term given to persistent anxiety. While both are treated in a similar fashion, the disorder is much more serious and requires long term and preventative treatments.

Prevention: Anxiety is a common side effect of many pharmaceuticals, so avoidance of prescription medications unless absolutely necessary will help in the prevention of anxiety. If taking anti-anxiety medication, additional herbal treatments should not be attempted.

Overuse of stimulants such as caffeine can also lead to adrenal exhaustion, which can in turn increases anxiety. If prone to anxiety, avoidance of these substances is an effective prevention method.

Treatments: Sometimes, excessive stress of other unavoidable lifestyle changes can lead to anxiety. For these cases, adaptogens are a great way to boost the body's ability to adapt to these changes without causing detrimental effects. Holy basil and astragalus are two common adaptogens, and both are also known to boost the immune system, which is often hindered during times of stress and increased emotions. New Chapter Organics produces a high quality holy basil supplement that is a favorite of mine.

Chamomile is a traditional remedy for anxiety in both adults and children. It also serves as a digestive aid, which offers benefits for the intestinal trouble that often accompanies anxiety. Chamomile is best taken as a warm herbal tea, and the quiet tea time also helps to bring about a calm feeling.

Kava kava contains kavalactones, which are compounds that work on the part of the brain that controls the nervous system and is especially responsible for the emotions. Kava does not cause addiction or tolerance with long term use, unlike many pharmaceuticals which generally require an increased dose to maintain therapeutic results. Kava can, however, cause a feeling of inebriation, so care should be taken to maintain the lowest necessary dose for therapeutic benefits, and individuals taking kava should avoid driving a vehicle or operating heavy machinery until they are more familiar with how their bodies tolerate the herb.

Appetite Loss

What is it? While loss of appetite may seem like a good thing to the perpetual dieter, it can actually be quite the health problem for many individuals, especially when it involves the appetite of a young child. Appetite loss or picky eating can lead to "failure to thrive" or other serious nutritional deficiencies. While it is certainly common for the average toddler to go through some phases of pickiness regarding their food, a significant decrease in appetite is nothing to shrug off.

Prevention: Many nutritional deficiencies can lead to lack of appetite, which often creates a downward spiral, as the lack of nutritional intake only leads to further nutritional deficiencies. Common culprits are zinc and iron. These deficiencies also lead to developmental problems, so this is an important issue to uncover and treat, if applicable. (Note: Iron supplementation can lead to overdose, so it is important to have a care provider confirm a suspected iron deficiency. For more information, see Anemia.)

It is important not to give way to the popular motherly advice "don't worry, he / she will eat when he / she gets hungry!" Many failure to thrive toddlers or young children simply do not feel hungry. Without an appetite, they will not eat because they do not get hungry! If a child regularly goes without eating, is losing weight (or not gaining weight) and seems to rarely ask for food or express hunger, this approach could be dangerous. Appetite can often return after nutritional deficiencies are addressed and herbal bitters are administered.

Treatments: If a nutritional deficiency exists, it is important to address that first. Supplements can be added to drinks if the child refuses to consume it as a tablet or in food.

Common herbal bitters that stimulate the appetite include orange peel, dandelion, fenugreek, yarrow, blessed thistle and coriander. Fenugreek can also lower blood sugar, so if that is a problem, it should not be added to a blend. Many blends go by the name "herbal bitters", so look for a child-safe blend that contains these and / or additional herbs.

Onions also help to stimulate the appetite, but consumption generally requires the individual to eat something first! If possible, the addition of onions to the diet can help increase the amount of food consumed.

Arthritis

What is it? Arthritis literally means "joint inflammation" and has also gone by the name degenerative joint disease. There are actually two main types of arthritis, rheumatoid and osteoarthritis, although osteoarthritis is currently ten times more common than rheumatoid.

Osteoarthritis is known as the "wear and tear" kind of arthritis. It is a chronic condition, characterized by the actual breaking down of the joints' cartilage. This allows the bones to rub together, which causes pain and loss of movement. There is no known cause or cure for osteoarthritis, but certain factors are generally accepted as playing a major role in determining who experiences arthritis.

Prevention: Considering that common treatments include weight control, diet and exercise, we can assume that these factors would also serve as effective prevention measures.

Treatments: There is some evidence that hormonal changes may accelerate or initiate arthritis, which may be why women are more likely to experience arthritis. The hormonal root causes can be treated with both milk thistle supplementation as a daily liver support and with an increase of foods rich in phytoestrogens. Milk thistle supplements should be standardized to contain 80% or more silymarin, which is the active compound in the herb.

There is also substantial evidence that Vitamin C and antioxidants can reduce the loss of cartilage and slow the progression of the disease. This reminds us once again to consume a healthy diet, rich in a wide variety of colorful foods, which offer an abundance of antioxidants.

By far, the most common natural remedy is glucosamine sulfate, which is a molecule of glucose and an amine in a chelated form. As many individuals age, glucosamine is naturally lost in the body, which causes the cartilage to lose its consistency. In trials, the benefits took as little as four weeks to appear. These benefits included both a reduction in pain and an increase in movement. While glucosamine is neither anti-inflammatory nor analgesic, it offers better long terms results than NSAIDs (non steroidal anti-inflammatory drugs) without the harmful side effects.

An anti-inflammatory blend by New Chapter Organics called Zyflamend is also highly effective at reducing the inflammation. Less inflammation results in less pain and more movement. The blend also offers antioxidants and nutrients that assist the body with detoxification.

The herb turmeric contains curcumin, an active compound that is a powerful anti-inflammatory that is effective at treating arthritis. General dose is 400mg curcumin / day.

Cayenne pepper contains a substance called capsaicin, which is applied topically and functions as an analgesic and anti-inflammatory. As a pepper extract, capsaicin can cause slight burning for some overly sensitive individuals. If that occurs, use should be discontinued. Creams should contain 0.25% to 0.75% capsaicin for optimal benefit.

Another traditional treatment for arthritis is ginger. Gingerol, one of the compounds in the herb, can inhibit the production of prostaglandins. Standard dose for this use is 10-20 drops of standard 1:5 tincture in water up to three times a day.

Recent trials show that a topical application of an arnica ointment helps to relieve pain with no side effects. When compared to conventional over the counter remedies, it offered much more benefit.

Arnica Infused Oil
Take 1 ounce of arnica (dried and cut) and place in an oven proof bowl. Add 10 ounces olive oil and place into the oven. The oven should have been preheated to 200 degrees, then turned off. Leave in the oven as it cools for 3-4 hours. Remove and leave at room temperature for an additional 4-5 hours. Strain the herbs out. To do this, cheesecloth, unbleached muslin or even a coffee filter work well. Pour the clean oil into a glass bottle and store at cool temperatures for the longest shelf life.

Athlete's foot
(Ringworm / Jock Itch)

What is it? Surprisingly, these three problems are all caused by the same common source: a fungal infection by the name of tinea. When it appears on the feet, it is termed tinea piedis or athlete's foot; on the groin or thigh it is termed tinea cruris or "jock itch" and elsewhere on the body it is tinea corporis or ringworm. An infection causes red, itchy skin and painful inflammation.

Prevention: Since the parasites that cause this infection grow in warm, dark and damp places, the best prevention is to eliminate these conditions from occurring together in the body. For example, we should ensure that our feet are covered when at a pool or other similar places and remember to remove or change socks after exercise or during hot, summery days.

The infection can be easily spread, so prompt and thorough hand washing after touching or scratching affected areas is a must.

Treatments: The best remedy for tinea infections is our multipurpose garlic oil. This oil offers many antifungal properties and is easy to obtain for topical use. Best of all, it is safe and gentle enough for little ones.

Chamomile also offers antifungal properties and is generally pretty easy to find in a conventional store. Small tea packets can be used to make a water infusion, which can be applied topically to the affected area. The stronger the tea, the more potent the application will be.

Another herb with antifungal properties is ginger. The best way to use ginger as a treatment is not to take it internally, rather to apply it topically directly to the affected area. Ginger tea can be made by steeping up to an ounce of ginger to a cup of boiling water. This brewed tea can be applied to the area with a washcloth several times a day.

Tea tree oil also offers beneficial properties, and is also applied topically. Like all essential oils, it is best to apply in a highly diluted form, especially when applying to children or sensitive areas of the body. Tea tree oil can be mixed in a 1:1 ratio with olive oil for topical application.

Autism

What is it? Autism is not a specific disorder, rather a spectrum of disorders that affect childhood development, social behaviors and overall health.

Prevention: At present, we have numerous theories as to what causes autism, but nothing solid in terms of prevention. We do know that autism is no longer considered to be genetic, since it has reached epidemic proportions, and there is no such thing as a genetic epidemic.

While we may not have something concrete to look for, the experts are beginning to reveal a number of potential causes in what is termed the multiple trigger theory. This suggests that there are actually numerous causes of autism and that each child has a predisposed breaking point, which determines exactly when these triggers actually trigger autism. This would fall right in line with the current treatment of autism, which includes first identifying which of the common imbalances are present and then treating those particular problems.

Treatments: There are numerous treatment options available to the family with an autistic child. While many of these are nothing more than urban legends, passed along from one mother to the next, changing as they go, much like the childhood game of telephone, many others are actually scientifically founded and can be highly successful at treating and even reversing autism for some children. Treating autism is too deep of a topic to adequately cover in this section, but some of the most commonly effective treatments include the GF/CF (gluten free and casein free) diet, avoidance of all artificial and processed foods, supplementation with certain amino acids and digestive enzymes to facilitate better absorption of nutrients, and ABA (applied behavioral analysis), which is the only currently FDA approved autism treatment. While any mother can easily pick up one of the numerous books on the subject and begin an assortment of autism therapies, it is important to remember that autism is a spectrum, not a precise disorder, so the treatments will be highly varied from individual to individual. What works effectively on one child may be totally useless for another.

Therefore, the best course of action for undertaking this type of treatment is to visit a DAN (Defeat Autism Now) physician. A licensed care provider with additional training on the latest therapies and studies can offer testing that will properly assess exactly which type of imbalance is present, helping to create an effective treatment plan for the individual. To find a DAN physician near you, go to www.autism.com and look for a local provider.

Backache

What is it? Backache is one of the most common concerns adults face today. In fact, it has been estimated that at some point in their lives, 80% of the population will experience backache so severe that it requires some sort of medical attention. Mainstream treatment previously consisted of rest and often surgery, but researchers have now convinced most physicians that these treatments are exactly the opposite of what our backs really need.

Instead, exercise actually reduces back pain. Experts project that up to 90% of those that experience chronic backaches do not regularly engage in exercise. Other non drug therapies that reduce back pain include yoga and chiropractic care.

Prevention: There are many causes for our backaches, including over exertion and lack of physical exercise. By using caution when lifting heavy items and ensuring plenty of daily exercise, we can often prevent intense backaches.

Treatments: Peppermint contains menthol, a common ingredient in many conventional preparations for backache and other similar pains. The essential oil, when diluted into olive oil or blended into a massage cream, makes a great solution for topical application, and when combined with massage can bring about speedy relief.

Capsaicum, an ingredient in red peppers, also brings about quick relief in a topical application. Creams containing 0.25% to 0.75% are readily available for topical application as a treatment for inflammation.

Chiropractic care is not an herbal treatment, but is generally indicated for all forms of backache. When I was nearing the end of the pregnancy of our third child, who just happened to be my largest child by nearly a pound and a half, chiropractic care was the only way I could get any relief from my chronic pain. Even when the source of the pain cannot be directly identified, chiropractic care can often locate the source, treat it effectively, and prevent reoccurrence.

Bedwetting

What is it? Technically speaking, bedwetting (nocturnal enuresis) can be common and is not considered to be problematic unless the child is 5 years or older. Most professionals do not recommend treatment prior to the age of 5, if not older. The wide range in which nighttime dryness is achieved is attributed to genetics, delayed development and sleep disorders.

Nonetheless, bedwetting can be embarrassing for a child, especially when he or she becomes old enough to begin requesting sleepovers. It can also cause sleepless nights, as parents are up to change linens in the middle of the night, and the laundry really begins to pile up!

Some experts have begun to detect a link between fathers that had a tendency to wet the bed and children that wet the bed. It is important to remember that staying dry all night is not a character flaw, but a developmental issue. Patience usually goes a long way with these children during such an embarrassing time.

Prevention: The best prevention for bedwetting is to limit the amount of fluids, especially sugary ones that a child drinks prior to bedtime. To ensure the body remains sufficiently hydrated during this adjustment, it is important to offer plenty of fluids during the morning and early afternoon.

There are also certain substances in the diet that can contribute to bedwetting for certain children. These include stimulants such as caffeine, hidden food sensitivities, artificial foods and underlying causes such as urinary tract infections or vaginal infections.

Treatments: Herbs that help to relax the CNS (Central Nervous System) can promote restful sleep and prevent bedwetting occurrences. This is best administered by establishing a routine that includes a special bedtime tea. Since we want to limit the fluids that the child takes in, we want to keep this to a six ounce cup and ensure the child has plenty of time to "potty" prior to bedtime.

Pumpkin seeds have also been used to successfully treat bedwetting. Germany's Commission E monographs list the dose as 10 g (roughly 1 T) a day. The seeds should be chewed well to maximize the absorption of the active amino acids and phytosterols.

Bites

(insect bites / stings)

What is it? Pests can attack throughout the year, but most of our common bug bites occur during the warmer months when we spend much of our time outdoors. An assortment of insects an be the cause of our bug bites, and it may be important to identify the insect in the event of an allergic reaction or potentially poisonous bite.

Prevention: Applying an essential oil blend to our bodies prior to exposure helps to prevent bug bites. Most popular insect repellants contain DEET, a chemical that quickly penetrates the body and brings long term effects that have not been proven to be safe.

Yet, many falsely believe that the alternative is to simply endure bugs and their biting. Not so! Many botanical oils effectively repel bugs, and many of them are more effective than DEET. These oils include basil, citronella, lemongrass and most citrus oils.

To create a homemade bug spray, combine any of these oils in a custom blend in a glass bottle. The citrus oils generally have a milder scent, so more should be used to balance the stronger basil and lemongrass odors. Blending essential oils is a fun and enjoyable task. I like to plan my blends by working with 1-2 drops of each oil at a time. They are blended, then left to mellow for a few hours. Once the desired blend is achieved, I make note of the exact ratio in the blend and then produce it in larger amount for regular use. For a bug spray, the essential oils blend should be diluted with olive or grapeseed oil so that it will not burn or irritate the skin. On average, 1 teaspoon of the oil blend should be diluted in 1 tablespoon of the olive or grapeseed oil.

Treatments: The first step is to check for any remaining insect parts that are in need of removal. Next, we want to observe for any potential allergic reactions, as that would often require immediate medical attention. Then we will have a better assessment of the situation, and we can proceed to treat at home.

For most bites, itching is the biggest problem, so an anti-inflammatory balm or salve is going to be ideal. Good options include calendula balms (such as the recipe below), chamomile salves and even plantain poultices. For intense itching, a warm bath with nourishing oats can bring about additional relief.

A dab of lavender essential oil blended with our balm or salve can add some antiseptic properties, and is often plenty to bring about relief.

Plantain is the classic herbalist's remedy for bug bites. It is well suited for this purpose, as it is a very common lawn weed, thus readily available in the outdoors. It is also an ingredient in many balms intended for bug bites or stings.

Garlic contains enzymes that break down the prostaglandins that the body produces in response to pain, so it would bring about pain relief when taken internally or applied topically directly to the affected area.

Calendula Balm
Materials include: 1/2 cup dried calendula petals (available in bulk at a health food store or from your garden; you may find it under it's nickname, marigold), 1 ounce beeswax, 1/2 cup olive oil, a sterile tin to hold your finished project.
Place the petals and oil into an oven proof dish. Preheat the oven to 200 degrees. Place the oil and herbs into the oven, then turn it off. Leave for 3-4 hours, then remove from the oven. It may need to cool for an hour or two on the counter. Once it is cool, strain out the herbs with cheesecloth. Add the beeswax to the remaining oil and put back into the oven (or you can use a microwave for this part.) Heat just until the beeswax is almost melted. Then you can take it out and stir until it is all melted and combined. Pour into your prepared tins and let sit 15-20 minutes until cool. This will make 2 tins of balm, about 2 ounces each.

Body Odor

What is it? Body odor is a dreaded situation for just about everybody. While we all envision ourselves as possessing a light, fresh scent around us, real life requires hard work and sweat, which often leads to unpleasant aromas. These scents often come from the underarms and feet, which are both prone to excessive sweating (or "glowing", as we called it growing up).

The underarm contains glands that are there throughout our lives, however just prior to puberty they begin to secrete an odorless liquid. If this liquid is not washed away within a few hours, bacteria begins to grow and omit a foul odor.

Prevention: Preventing body odor is a real problem for many natural minded individuals, since most deodorants contain aluminum, which is a neurotoxin. However, there are many alternatives to mainstream deodorants, and some individuals choose to alternate between the mainstream products during especially stressful times and hot steamy days, and the alternatives for the milder and cooler days.

Body odor can also be caused by a zinc deficiency, sluggish liver, constipation and / or parasites. Attention to healthy dietary habits can play a key role in reducing these factors.

Treatments: Sage helps not only to fight off bacteria on the skin, but also to actually inhibit sweating, much like our conventional antiperspirants and deodorants. Sage oil should not be applied directly to the skin, but ground sage can be blended with baking soda, cornstarch and rosemary to make a odor fighting body powder. To make your own: combine 1/2 cup each baking soda and cornstarch (or tapioca powder) with 1 tablespoon each powdered sage and rosemary.

Fennel is a popular digestive aid, but has some additional benefits for those that choose to use it. It seems that these digestive actions help to regulate certain types of bad breath and body odor that originate in the intestines. This can help to treat the problem from the inside out.

Homemade Sage Deodorant
2 cups apple cider vinegar
1/2 cup sage (cut and sifted)
1/4 cup rosemary
2 sticks cinnamon
Combine in a glass canning jar. Cap and shake well to disperse contents evenly. Place near a sunny window and shake again 1-2 times a day for 21 days. Strain and store in a clearly labeled bottle. To use: apply with cotton ball to underarms 3-4 times a day. Here's a quick tip to make natural deodorants more effective: As the body "glows", the moisture will wash away the deodorant, so reapplication should occur every 3-4 hours or when moisture is felt.

Breast Infection
(mastitis)

What is it? Mastitis simply means breast infection, and is usually a result of a clogged duct. When the body produces breast milk, it flows through ducts, or small little tunnels in the breasts. When these ducts become engorged, which often happens during weaning, or when baby has not eaten for an extended period of time, or when they are physically constricted, such as compression from a wire lined bra or lying on the breast when it is full, the stagnant milk can quickly become infected.

When this happens, there is usually a red area on the painful side of the breast, and a lump can often be felt. Symptoms come on suddenly and include fatigue, fever, chills, nausea and flu-like symptoms. If treated quickly, the infection can often clear up just as quickly as it came, but if not, it can lead to a breast abscess, which requires medical intervention.

Prevention: Mastitis can be prevented by ensuring that the new mother obtains plenty of rest and drinks plenty of fluids. Dehydration and fatigue can both lead to clogged ducts, which lead to mastitis. When a duct does become clogged, prompt attention can usually prevent mastitis as well. Breastfeeding professionals suggest aligning the baby's chin with the clogged duct while nursing. This often requires a bit of imagination at coming up with positions to nurse, but usually eliminates the problem within a couple of nursing sessions.

Treatments: Garlic is effective at treating mastitis, especially when combined with echinacea. For this use, it is usually best to stick with the supplement form of garlic, unless mommy feels up to consuming several fresh cloves! Likewise, an echinacea / goldenseal or Oregon grape root blend is a good antibacterial remedy for a breast infection.

During an infection, it is important to stay hydrated. An eight ounce glass of water should be taken every hour until the infection has cleared. For topical relief, warm wet compresses can be very effective at reducing the pain and discomfort. For additional anti-inflammatory properties, an infusion of calendula or chamomile can be warmed for the compress.

Breastfeeding
(milk supply)

What is it? Breastfeeding may be the best way of providing nourishment to a growing baby, but that does not mean it is trouble free for every mommy and baby team that choose it. Unfortunately, a breastfeeding relationship can occasionally experience difficulties such as poor milk supply or mastitis (breast infection). Usually, these challenges can be overcome with some hard work and patience, but they can often be difficult to face with a new baby to care for. For more serious problems, such as extremely low milk supply or latching issues, it is best to schedule an in person visit with an IBCLC (International Board Certified Lactation Consultant) for help and troubleshooting, then team up with your local chapter of LLL (La Leche League) for encouragement and ongoing assistance.

Prevention: The best way to prevent most breastfeeding problems is to nurse early and often! Milk supply is based on the principle of supply and demand. Unfortunately, many baby "experts" advocate strict feeding schedules for baby, which can lead to breastfeeding disasters. It is important to remember that the medical community at large does not advocate such restricted feedings, and researchers support feeding babies "on demand" for at least the first 6 months of life. This concept is supported by the World Health Organization as well as many other respected medical organizations. "On demand" means no "parent initiated" feeding schedules, the baby eats when he or she is hungry or every 2-3 hours during the day and no longer than 4 hours at night (initially).

This frequent nursing pattern not only helps to establish a healthy milk supply, it helps to prevent failure to thrive babies and helps to prevent the baby from going too long between meals, which in turn lead to mastitis. When we sit down to feed our little ones, we enjoy the added benefit of a "forced" break from our days, which helps mom to focus and rest as the beneficial calming hormones are released, having been triggered by the letdown of mommy's milk. The design behind the nourishment of our babies is a wonderful creation indeed!

Treatments: For poor milk supply, certain herbs called galactagogues are known to increase the milk production. Fenugreek is probably the most common galactogogue, and has a history that dates back to biblical times, but it also contains side effects that should be taken into consideration. For babies or mommies that may be prone to hypoglycemia, fenugreek is not recommended. Otherwise, it can be easily brewed into a tea and consumed throughout the day or powdered and applied directly to the breasts topically, which is the traditional use. The properties of the herb are absorbed directly through the skin and can provide reliable results. Fenugreek also gives the milk a maple syrup odor, which is harmless. (Don't take fenugreek during pregnancy!)

When I meet with clients, however, fenugreek is not my herb of choice, instead I prefer to discuss milk thistle and blessed thistle. Both thistles also offer reliable results, but without the potential side effects, and with additional liver boosting properties, which provide additional benefits for both mama and baby. Milk thistle should always be standardized to contain 80% or more silymarin, which is the active compound in the herb.

Many mothers are given strict instructions by well meaning individuals that usually involve restricting the diet to consist of only bland foods to avoid giving baby "gas". This old wives tale is not only false, it can lead to frustration in the brestfeeding relationship, as the mother eventually tires from having to avoid all of her favorite foods. In reality, the herb garlic, both as a supplement and liberal addition to the diet, has been shown to cause babies to attach ("latch on") much better, to stay on the breast longer, and to drink more milk at each feeding. This increase in demand leads to an increase in supply.

Bronchitis

What is it? The term bronchitis refers to inflammation of the mucus lining of the bronchial tubes. These tubes carry air from the trachea to the lungs. The inflammation can be a result of a viral or bacterial infection and, as it progresses leads to an increase in mucus production, which produces a deep and wet sounding cough.

Other symptoms include difficult or painful breathing, persistent coughing, yellow or green mucus production and fever. This can all result in fatigue and an overall achy feeling.

While the inflammation usually clears up in 7-10 days, the cough can linger for weeks, although it should generally become more and more infrequent during this time.

Prevention: Smoking can make an individual more prone to bronchitis and can slow the healing process, so avoidance of smoke, both first and second hand is crucial for avoidance of the inflammation.

Research also shows that common air pollutants such as formaldehyde can irritate the airways, increasing the likelihood of bronchitis. One surprising way to reduce the toxin levels in the home (which is notorious for polluted air) is to increase the number of indoor plants. Studies show that plants such as ferns actually clean the air, making it safer to breathe.

Additionally, consumption of a whole foods diet, rich in fresh fruits and vegetables is useful in the prevention of all viral and bacterial infections. Care when exposed to illness, and immune boosting herbs when appropriate also aid in preventing bronchitis.

Treatments: Wild cherry bark is a classic treatment for coughing, especially while the cough is still dry. It should not be taken in excessive doses or for extended periods of time, but when taken appropriately, it is safe enough even for children. Ideally, wild cherry bark is taken in a cough syrup or antiviral blend of herbs, so the herb is combined with other herbs, resulting in an even lower intake of wild cherry bark, preventing overdose. My personal favorite is Herbs for Kids Cherry Bark Blend.

Mullein offers expectorant properties, which helps to break up phlegm so that it can be coughed up. It also helps to soothe the throat and stops the muscle spasms that trigger coughing.

Horehound, an herb that is approved by Germany's Commission E for bronchial complaints. Old fashioned horehound candies make excellent herbal cough drops. The trick is to check the ingredient list to ensure they actually contain horehound and not just flavoring.

Research shows that as magnesium levels in the body decrease, the incidence of respiratory disease increases. Considering that many individuals are deficient in magnesium, supplementation is a great treatment for those prone to respiratory infections.

Slippery elm bark helps to coat the throat, reducing irritation and decreasing the intensity of the coughing spells. These actions are due to the mucilage content of the plant. To obtain these benefits, the herb must be able to coat the throat, so extracts or encapsulated herbs will not work.

Steam treatments are also classically used to help with the intensity of nighttime coughing. When eucalyptus or peppermint oils are added, they can help relax the airways, promoting clearer breathing. Both oils are highly potent and should be diluted prior to use with at least equal parts of olive oil, if not more. Neither oil should be diffused near the face.

Bruises

What is it? A bruise is a broken blood vessel beneath intact skin. They turn shades of blue, red and green, look awful and often feel as bad as they look! While young children generally prefer a bandage for such painful situations, the body generally heals itself with bruises requiring no further treatment.

Prevention: There is not much that we can do to prevent bruises, Life is necessarily full of obstacles and clumsy accidents are just a part of it.

However, nutritional deficiencies can often lead to more frequent or common bruising, so a healthy balanced diet actually prevents bruising for many individuals.

Treatments: Anti-inflammatory balms and salves can be beneficial at speeding the healing time for a bruise. A balm can be made at home with dried calendula or chamomile or can be found fairly easily at any health food store.

Additional intake of Vitamin C has also been shown to decrease the duration of the discoloration. This can be as simple as boosting the fruits and vegetables rich in the nutrient or adding a Vitamin C rich multivitamin or supplement to the diet.

Arnica provides analgesic, anti-inflammatory and antiseptic properties that can actually reduce the healing time of the bruise. Ointments and oils should be applied topically, but arnica should not be used internally or on broken skin.

Comfrey contains allantoin, which helps to reduce inflammation and heal the bruise on the cellular level. It should not be taken internally, but topical applications of oils or creams are beneficial and have even received the approval of Germany's Commission E.

Burns

What is it? A burn is a common childhood accident, but can often be serious enough to warrant immediate medical treatment. We categorize burns by sorting them into three stages. The milder burns (stage one and some stage two) can be easily treated at home with comforting remedies.

A mild burn is one in which only the outer layer of skin has been affected. The skin will be red and occasionally blisters, swelling and pain will also be present. If a large part of the hands, feet, face, groin, buttocks or major joints are affected, additional help should be sought immediately, as this often indicates a more serious burn is present.

Prevention: Like many household accidents, there are not any additional measures we can undertake to reduce the occurrence. Common sense measures should always be taken in the home when children are present as their natural curiosity can often lead to dangerous accidents.

Treatments: Drinking water is actually quite beneficial at treating burns both at home and in the case of a more serious burn under medical treatment. Many nutrients also speed would healing, including Vitamins A, B complex and C, zinc and essential fatty acids.

Topically, Echinacea is known to speed wound healing and can be applied in a compress made by brewing dried herbs into a tea or blending an extract with some water. Anti-inflammatory herbs such as calendula and chamomile can be applied topically in a similar manner.

Aloe vera gel has been used medicinally since the Egyptians and is beneficial for soothing inflammation, reducing pain and fighting bacteria. It also helps the burn to heal faster.

Lavender essential oil can be applied topically to a burn undiluted. Normally we never apply an essential oil to the skin undiluted, but lavender is one of the rare exceptions. The oil speeds wound healing and is especially effective on burns. To use, dab a few drops onto the affected area with a cotton swab or ball. With young children or those sensitive to lavender, the oil can be diluted with equal parts olive oil.

The area should be kept sterile, to prevent infection, but plenty of fresh air also helps speed the healing process. For adults this is not as difficult, but it is difficult to keep a child's unbandaged wound clean, so sterile bandages might be in order. If an infection is suspected, antiseptic herbs such as goldenseal and Oregon grape root can be applied by powdering the dried herb and dabbing the powder directly onto the affected area.

Canker Sores

What is it? Canker sores are small lesions that develop in the soft tissues of the mouth (also known as aphthous ulcers). Prime locations include the area under the tongue, inside of the cheeks and at the base of the gums. They are not contagious, but can be painful, especially during mealtime.

Prevention: There are many probable causes of canker sores, including immune system disorders, certain bacteria, hormonal shifts, stress, certain nutritional deficiencies, and even oral hygiene products containing sodium laurel sulfate. The most common cause, however, is a food allergy or sensitivity.

Therefore, like most of our common health problems, canker sores are best prevented by a healthy diet, with a wide assortment of whole foods, healthy stress responses, and a naturally minded lifestyle.

Treatments: When canker sores cannot be avoided, they will generally go away on their own in 1-2 weeks. However, herbal medicine can certainly help speed that along.

Myrrh is approved by Germany's Commission E as a treatment for oral inflammation. Powdered myrrh can be found in capsules at a health food store, and opened to apply directly to the lesion. According to Dr. James Duke, the myrrh is effective in large part to the tannin content, so other foods rich in tannins would also be beneficial.

Oregon grape root is effective at healing wounds and infections, including oral lesions. Many natural mouthwashes feature Oregon grape root (or goldenseal), making it an effective treatment and prevention method for canker sores and halitosis (bad breath).

Licorice is a fast remedy for many oral sores, including both canker sores and cold sores. In one study, a licorice mouthwash brought improvement in as little as 24 hours, and complete relief by 3 days to 75% of participants.

Canker Sore Potion

This gel brings together some of the best herbs for canker sores. To use, apply a small dab directly to the sore with a cotton swab. (Not intended for pregnant or lactating mommies.)

1 teaspoon beeswax
2 tablespoons olive oil
1 teaspoon Chamomile extract
1 teaspoon Oregon Grape Root extract
1 teaspoon Licorice extract
1 teaspoon Gotu kola extract

1 teaspoon Echinacea extract
Combine the olive oil and beeswax in a small jar. Microwave or warm over low heat until the beeswax is just melted. Add the extracts, stirring constantly to blend well. Pour mixture into a sterile metal tin to cool.

Carpal Tunnel Syndrome

What is it? Before the era of computers and tiny cell phones, very few individuals had even heard of carpal tunnel syndrome. Our constant repetitive and rapid use of the fingers on tiny keyboards has led to a type of trauma to the nerves. More specifically, it is the compression of the median nerve, which passes through the "carpal tunnel" or bones and ligaments of the wrist. It is a "wear and tear" type injury, that results in swelling, pain, weakness and a pins and needles sensation.

Women are more prone to carpal tunnel syndrome than men, and obviously, anyone in a career that requires constant repetitive movement of the hands or fingers will be more likely to suffer. This can include not only those of us that spend our days in front of the computer screen, but hair stylists, seamstresses, and carpenters.

Prevention: The best way to prevent carpal tunnel syndrome is to exercise the wrists and fingers between working and during frequent breaks. This helps combat the repetitive motion, massaging the area to prevent compression.

There is also sufficient evidence that a deficiency in vitamin B complex and C increase the chance of carpal tunnel syndrome, so supplementation with these nutrients can help reduce those chances. Considering that carpal tunnel syndrome is inflammatory related, antioxidants, a diet rich in fruits and vegetables, and sufficient omega 3 fatty acids would also provide preventative benefits.

Treatments: Turmeric contains anti-inflammatory properties that can reduce the swelling and pressure, which lessens the pain. Considering what a common culinary herb turmeric is, the liberal use of the herb in the diet would play a key role in both prevention and treatment.

Gingko helps to increase the blood flow, which would also stop inflammation in the hands, reducing swelling. This increased blood flow also boosts memory and cognitive function, so it would be my herb of choice, if I were to face carpal tunnel syndrome.

Whole foods often offer substantial benefits as medicinal agents. Pineapple and papaya both contain bromelain, which is a protein dissolving enzyme that reduces inflammation in the body. This reduction leads to decreased swelling and pain. Studies show that very large amounts of the substance can be taken safely, so if neither food suits your taste buds, bromelain supplements are available at most health food stores.

Capsaicum, a compound found in cayenne and red peppers is also commonly used in both botanical and conventional medicine as a treatment for swelling and inflammation in the hands. More popular in arthritis treatments, the extract also provides benefits for those with carpal tunnel syndrome. Ointments or creams should contain 0.25%-0.75% capsaicum content.

Cellulite

What is it? Cellulite is a French term that refers to the stores of fatty tissue just below the surface of the skin that is due to weakened connective tissue commonly found in women. This leads to a dimply appearance on the thighs and hips.

Prevention: Proper nutrition and exercise have been beneficial in preventing cellulite. Studies show us that thin women and athletic women have little to no cellulite. Of course we want to caution against excess in this area, which can lead to other health problems, but a nutritious diet coupled with plenty of exercise can generally assist with preventing cellulite.

Treatments: Many cosmetic products will claim to have the ability to reduce cellulite, or at least the appearance of cellulite, but few have actually proven to have that ability. Fortunately, there are botanical remedies that have held up to rigorous trials.

Weleda makes a highly effective oil product called Birch Cellulite Oil, which has been clinically shown to reduce cellulite when used over a few weeks. This oil is a personal favorite of mine.

Gotu kola has also been shown to be effective at strengthening tissues, which lead to a reduction of both varicose veins and cellulite. It generally takes three months of oral intake for results to be seen.

Cholesterol

What is it? The term cholesterol refers to a substance that is carried through the blood on carrier molecules known as lipoproteins. There are different types of lipoproteins, low density (LDL), high density (HDL) and very low density (VLDL).

High cholesterol (hypercholesterolemia) is generally diagnosed with a total count over 200, but modern experts are beginning to concern themselves more with the ratio than the actual numbers. Following this line of thought, ideal LDL ("bad") numbers should be close to or less than 130, while ideal HDL ("good") numbers should be close to or above 35.

Prevention: Like the majority of our modern common ailments, high cholesterol is often caused by poor diet and inactivity. The best way to prevent high cholesterol is to gradually change to a whole foods diet, low in animal fats and high in plant foods, and make sure the body gets plenty of activity or exercise.

Treatments: Modern treatments aimed at lowering cholesterol numbers are often laden with undesired (and dangerous) side effects, such as liver damage. In fact, long term trials do not show an increase in life expectancy with these drugs, only a change in the type of health problem experienced.

Natural treatments, however, are also effective at reducing the numbers and altering the ratios, but with the added benefits of antioxidants and assorted whole food nutrients. These treatments typically reduce the overall numbers by 50-75 mg/dl within 2-3 months, but will usually take longer to bring about ideal numbers and ratios in those with especially high cholesterol at the start.

Garlic is one of my favorite cholesterol treatments. While the German Commission E recommends fresh cloves, the capsules are more socially acceptable, and according to research, just as effective. Kyolic has some great blends designed especially for altering the ratios and reducing the numbers.

Another proven, yet seldom used, remedy is naturally occurring fiber. Studies show great results at lowering total cholesterol, and especially at reducing LDL numbers, but many individuals avoid this remedy due to its sheer simplicity. Great high fiber foods include carrots, celery, beans, just about any fresh green, and the old fashioned remedy from the 1980s, whole oats. To fully enjoy the benefits of added dietary fiber, keep a close eye out for the cholesterol in the diet, especially animal sources. I have personally seen many clients undertake a vegan or (low animal fat) vegetarian diet for 3-4 months to get their cholesterol under control, then maintain their success with a high plant food / low animal fat diet and plenty of exercise.

Cold / Flu

What is it? These two twins of the winter months are usually termed interchangeably, but the two are actually drastically different. This might be why those that choose to obtain the flu vaccine are often surprised when they continue to get sick during the winter months!

Both are viral infections of the upper respiratory tract, and both are treated with similar remedies (which is why they fall under the same heading), but the symptoms offer insight as to their true identity.

A cold carries with it a mild cough, achy feeling, sore throat and stuffy or even runny nose. Sneezing and watery eyes are also common. It generally does not involve a fever or headache, and will run its course in 7-10 days, but will cause mild fatigue during that timeframe.

The flu, on the other hand, brings a more intense cough, achy feeling, headache and fever, sometimes a high fever. This viral infection lasts much longer, generally around 12-14 days and will often bring a sore throat and stuffy nose, but usually not sneezing and watery eyes.

Another tell tale distinction is the manner in which these infections begin. Generally speaking, a cold will come on slowly, over the course of a day or two, while the flu often comes on suddenly, often within a couple of hours.

Prevention: Both viral illnesses are prevented with good common sense prevention measures and a healthy diet. This includes frequent hand washing, especially during situations when increased exposure is likely.

Antibacterial agents such as hand soaps, cleaning supplies and many hand sanitizers are not effective at preventing viral illness, since they are designed to kill bacteria. Evidence shows that hand washing with regular soap and warm water is still the best way of reducing our exposure. Other common sense tips include keeping our own family members at home when they are ill and encouraging our friends to do the same, cleaning doorknobs and other commonly touched items with antiviral essential oil products, with oils such as eucalyptus, lavender, tea tree and lemon, or even spraying or diffusing these oils throughout the home when a crowd is expected.

Additionally, I find it a strange coincidence that the winter viral season often begins right around the time Halloween candy is distributed and often ends right after New Year's or Valentine's Day. During these closely set holidays, we are prone to "indulge" in extra sugary treats. Sugar products lower our immune systems by up to 40% for up to 4 hours after intake. When we combine a decrease in immune function with close indoor interaction with other individuals (and their assorted "germs") and other holiday stresses, it really is difficult to wonder why we become ill every year around this time. In our home, we combat this with additional immune support such as astragalus root supplements or elderberry extract. We also limit our sugary intake to situations when we are not experiencing increased exposure to illness, and make sure our bodies are well stocked with nutrients to fight off illness.

Vitamin D is a common deficiency in the winter months, and studies show supplementation with a good whole foods multivitamin can reduce the occurrence of viral infections. Nordic Berries by Nordic Naturals is a favorite in the Hawkins' home during this time of year!

Treatments: When prevention fails us and we find ourselves "coming down" with a cold or the flu, all is not lost. We can still support our body's natural functions with natural remedies that are shown to reduce the intensity and duration of these common illnesses. Our personal family experience is that, with proper nutrition, avoidance of sugars, and plenty of rest and herbal remedies a cold generally passes within 2-3 days.

Echinacea is the most common cold / flu remedy. It is best used at the first onset of symptoms, not before. It is clinically proven to reduce the duration of the common cold and can cause a reduction in the intensity of symptoms.

Immune boosters, such as astragalus and elderberry should be continued through the cold or flu for optimal benefits. Elderberry syrups by Sambucol or Herbs for Kids are staples in the Hawkins' home and can offer great additional benefits for a cold.

Garlic is useful in both supplemental form and as an addition to the diet. It boosts the immune system, helping ward off both viral and bacterial infections. Fresh garlic is best, and studies show that if it must be cooked, the beneficial properties can be preserved by letting the cut garlic sit out for 10 or more minutes after cutting. Odorless supplements are also available for adults. These also have very mild blood thinning properties, which should be taken into consideration for those taking or avoiding blood thinners. If in doubt, contact a professional for more details.

Essential oils can help relieve the symptoms of a stuffy nose, providing a feeling of clearer breathing. Beneficial oils include eucalyptus, peppermint and spearmint. While these oils are extremely potent and should not be applied to the skin, a single drop or two can be blended with a teaspoon of carrier oil (olive is a great choice) and added to a warm bath, shower or even simply diffused into a room. The minty oils will also help alleviate any associated headaches.

Adults can take advantage of the ancient practice of nasal cleansing. This saline rinse helps to clear the sinus passages, allowing clearer breathing and preventing the stuffy nose feeling. For those prone to sinus infections, a blend of antibacterial extracts can be added to the saline solution to cleanse the area, preventing or treating infections. Herbs such as echinacea, Oregon grape root and goldenseal are often used for this purpose.

Cold Sores / Fever Blisters

What is it? Cold sores or fever blisters are caused by one of the herpes simplex viruses, but are not the same type of infections that cause genital herpes. These sores generally appear within a week after exposure and can usually last about 3 weeks at each outbreak. The virus lies dormant in the nervous system and additional outbreaks are triggered by many causes, including stress, decreased immune function, menstruation, fevers and viral infections.

The average cold sore goes through six stages at each outbreak, which averages 10 days. First, a tingling sensation appears on the affected area. It may even be slightly itchy. Next, the area may begin to turn reddish or begin to swell. Finally, the blister begins to appear. Each of these stages usually last around 24 hours. By the fourth day, the blister(s) is painful and begins to form a crust, which hardens. Unfortunately, this is when most individuals begin to seek treatment, which is after the outbreak has progressed significantly. By the tenth day, the crust falls off and all that is left is a reddened spot on the lip. Depending on the individual and the severity of the outbreak, these stages can take up to three weeks to be complete.

Prevention: Since the virus that causes cold sores lies dormant in the body, prevention revolves around preventing the outbreaks. Increasing the immune function and consuming a whole foods diet, especially during times of stress, are crucial to preventing cold sores. Additionally, treatment should begin at the first sign of tingling, instead of waiting for the full blown blister to erupt. This can prevent the outbreak from progressing through the stages, or hasten them along.

Treatments: By far, the best treatment for a cold sore is lemon balm, also known by its Latin name, *Melissa*. Lemon balm contains antiviral properties that have been clinically shown to reduce the size and severity of the outbreak by preventing healthy cells from becoming infected. A cream should contain at least 1% lemon balm extract and can be applied 5 times a day. This is a great ointment to keep on hand and apply to the skin immediately after experiencing the tingling sensation that signals the start of an outbreak.

Likewise, licorice offers many antiviral properties and reduces the duration of the outbreak by protecting healthy cells. Licorice makes a great addition to a topical ointment, but is not well suited for internal consumption with something as mild as a cold sore. Before taking it internally, be sure to look through the contraindications listed in the back.

Mullein helps to fight off the herpes virus and soothe irritated skin. It can be taken internally (30 drops of tincture every 4 waking hours) or applied topically to soothe irritation. One to two drops directly on the affected area is ideal.

Echinacea is an immune booster that works when taken after the onset of an infection. By taking it right at the beginning of the tingling sensation, it can effectively help fight off the infection.

Garlic is also well suited to any viral infection as it can increase the immune system and is easy to add to the diet. It can be applied topically for direct contact with the virus, but is usually used internally while one of our other remedies are applied directly onto the affected area.

Many essential oils offer antiviral properties. Tea tree and lavender are two of the most common oils, but clove has also been shown to provide powerful antiviral activity in trials, especially against the herpes virus. While the oils cannot be applied directly to the skin, one drop of any of the three can be blended with a teaspoon of olive oil and applied to the area with a cotton swab. Essential oils should never be taken internally.

Colic

What is it? Colic is the catch all term applied to persistent crying between the ages of three weeks and three months of age, although any experienced mama can verify that colic is not limited to these ages! The term actually comes from a Greek work referring to the small intestines, and many experts believe that intestinal problems often contribute to this unexplainable crying.

Prevention: One of the most common causes of infant crying is hunger. Experts inform us that newborns should never go longer than 3 hours during the day or 4 hours at night without a meal. Not only does this assure their little tummies stay well fed, it helps mom establish a healthy milk supply, ensuring the breastfeeding relationship can continue through any tough times.

Sometimes new babies will also "cluster feed", which means they might nurse every half hour or so for 2-3 hours at a time. During a growth spurt, babies might need to eat as often as every hour or two for a couple of days. All of this is perfectly normal. Just as our eating habits change from day to day, depending on how much energy we need or have used, so do a growing baby's.

This is certainly not to imply that all crying is due to hunger. Babies use crying as their main form of communication, which can mean their diaper is dirty, they are hot or cold, they are uncomfortable, or simply tired. Wearing the baby in a sling also helps to relieve crying, providing a safe and secure place for baby to snuggle up and sleep or simply bask in mommy's love.

When those measures fail, true colic might be the culprit. For these cases, treatment measures would be applicable.

Treatments: Studies show us that the common infant drops do very little to actually relieve colic in babies. What does help, however, is an infant blend of probiotics. At birth and shortly after, babies' tummies begin to develop what we call "intestinal flora" which is the combination of bacteria and yeasts in the intestines. Just like adults, when the ratio of beneficial microbes is altered, intestinal problems can crop up. When baby is born by cesarean or offered antibiotics at birth, both common practices in modern childbirth, the ratio can be altered, providing a need for supplementation with an infant blend of probiotics. One of my favorite brands is Udo's Choice by Flora Health, which is available at most health food stores or websites.

Additionally, a centuries old remedy is now becoming readily available at mainstream stores. Gripe water is a blend containing fennel and organic ginger, both of which are approved by Germany's Commission E as a treatment for intestinal troubles, including cramping and gas.

Conjunctivitis

What is it? Conjunctivitis, better known as pink eye, is an infection or inflammation of the transparent membrane that lines the eyelid and part of the eyeball. It is most commonly caused by a viral or bacterial infection, which makes the appearance of the blood vessels appear larger giving the eye a pink look. Other symptoms include discharge from the eye and blurry vision. Pink eye is highly contagious and can be transmitted for up to 7-14 days after the onset of symptoms.

Prevention: The best way to prevent pink eye is to avoid children that have it, since it is such a highly contagious infection. It is also important to remind our children to keep their fingers and hands out of their eyes, as well as to keep their eye products (especially make up) to themselves.

Treatments: One of the most effective ways to receive immediate relief from the symptoms is to apply a warm compress directly to the affected area. (Take care to keep the eye closed during this, as well as utilize common sense to avoid burns.)

A popular and effective herbal treatment for the infection and / or inflammation is aptly called eyebright. Not only does eyebright offer anti-inflammatory properties, it helps to fight off any infection that may be present. To use, squirt a couple of drops of the extract onto a warm washcloth and follow the preceding directions for a compress.

Berry leaves (blackberry or raspberry) also offer astringent properties that can help to decrease redness and the microbial actions of goldenseal or Oregon grape root can also help fight infection. These can be taken internally to fight infection from the inside out.

Constipation

What is it? Constipation is the term used for a bowel movement that is hard, compact, and difficult to pass. As one of the most common gastric complaints, Americans spend roughly $725 million annually on over the counter constipation relief aids.

The average individual should aim for one "output" for each "input", but most individuals fall short of that goal. As the digestion process occurs, our intestines absorb fluids from the waste as it is formed. When our waste sits too long in the intestines, more liquid is absorbed, which leads to hard and compact stools as well as the re-absorption of toxins from our waste. Other factors can also lead to constipation including a lack of fiber, intake of dairy products, certain medications, changes to daily routine, and even ignoring the urge to "go".

Prevention: Constipation can usually be prevented by ensuring the diet has plenty of fiber to bulk up the stool and keep things moving along at a regular pace. Ideal daily fiber intake is 25-40g, but the National Institute of Health estimates that the average American only consumes 12-18g. The best way to ensure plenty of fiber is to consume plenty of fresh fruits, veggies and whole grains in the diet.

Another great measure is to ensure the body remains well hydrated. My general rule of thumb is to divide the body weight in half, then change the "pounds" to "ounces" and make that my daily goal. For example: An individual that weighs 150 pounds would aim for 75 ounces of water daily.

Childhood constipation is also common as a result of potty training. Out of performance anxiety or outright fear, many children will hold it in as long as they can to avoid having to use the toilet. This is a good time for encouragement and patience, as their very real fears may seem petty to us grown ups that are familiar with the toilet and its functions.

Treatments: In many cases, the best treatment is to change the diet to include more fiber. If the body is not accustomed to sufficient fiber, this change should occur slowly, to prevent uncomfortable gas and bloating.

Gentle digestive aids include chamomile, ginger and fennel. These can often provide enough assistance to relieve mild constipation, and would assist with stronger remedies for more stubborn constipation. One of the bet ways to take advantage of these herbs is through a classic herbal tea. These flavors are strong, so those that prefer mild foods might not enjoy the remedy, but the additional water helps add hydration, which is often useful with constipation.

Many conventional laxatives contain psyllium husks as the active ingredient, however they also contain other ingredients that are not recommended. Instead, the same benefit can be obtained from a herbal psyllium capsule or even by adding the nutty tasting fiber directly to a green salad or other meal. Smaller amounts can be given to children, but the key with any herbal laxative is to offer minimal doses. As little as a half a teaspoon makes a good starting point, and the remedy can be continued every few hours until the bowels move.

Flax is another effective, yet mild laxative. Ground flaxseeds offer plenty of fiber to bring about relief, and can be easily tossed into a smoothie or bowl of cereal. Flax is also a great source of omega 3 fatty acids, which are usually deficient in individuals that consume the average diet.

For more difficult cases, cascara sagreda is a reliable laxative. It is usually considered too strong for children, and I recommend using it only as a last resort, but provides consistent results when used appropriately. While cascara is reported as having no potential for dependency in professional literature, I still always recommend a minimal dose for a minimal timeframe, to avoid any possibilities.

Croup

What is it? Croup is a common childhood disease, most frequently observed during the colder months. Children between the ages of three months and three years are most likely to develop croup, which identifies itself by an easily recognizable and harsh cough, resembling that of a seal, which presents itself more often at night. The cough occurs as a result of inflammation around the vocal cords, which can lead to hoarseness. It is highly contagious, usually caused by a virus.

Prevention: Prevention for croup is similar to the prevention measures we take for other winter viral illnesses, such as colds and coughs. A reduction in sugar intake, increased awareness of hand washing and other hygienic practices, and supplementation with immune boosting herbs such as astragalus, elderberry extract and garlic are all great prevention measures. For more details, be sure to flip back to the cold / flu section and review the prevention measures listed there.

Treatments: Most cases of viral croup can easily be treated at home, although if the voice is muffled or the child has difficulty swallowing saliva, a bacterial infection may be present and a trip to the family physician is warranted.

The classic home treatment of a shower steam is made more effective with the addition of eucalyptus essential oil. This oil is very potent and should never be applied directly onto the skin, but a single drop or two can be added to a teaspoon or two of olive oil to make a gentle remedy.

This oil is added to the bottom of the shower so that it can be diffused into the air and inhaled, providing clearer breathing.

Chamomile tea offers anti-inflammatory properties and can be beneficial for children that are old enough to drink other fluids, although breastfeeding babies should be getting plenty of breastmilk for the powerful immune boosting benefits.

Other immune boosting herbs should be continued for additional assistance as the body fights the virus, but be sure to take the age of the child into consideration before administering remedies.

Cradle Cap

What is it? Cradle cap is an inflammatory rash generally found on the scalp of babies, but can sometimes spread to the face or even other areas of the body. This rash is actually a secretion from the skin that forms a crusty scale like effect. It usually appears during the early weeks and clears up on its own within the first year, although some children seem to experience cradle cap that continues well into the second or even third year.

Contrary to popular thought, cradle cap is not caused by poor hygiene and is not an infection. The cause is actually unknown, but we do know it is painless and generally does not cause discomfort.

Prevention: As there is no known cause for cradle cap, there is no reliable prevention that can be taken. While the rash is not caused by poor hygiene, it can be worsened by infrequent washing of the scalp. Most babies do not need to be bathed more than 2-3 times per week, and more often could prove to be detrimental to their sensitive skin, but gently cleansing the scalp 2-3 times a week with the regular bath can help reduce the severity of cradle cap.

Treatments: The most common treatment is to apply baby oil to the scalp. Many experts now disagree with this theory for the same reasons we promote oil free cleansers for those with acne. However, when we consider that oil actually dissolves oil, an herbal oil treatment (with anti-inflammatory herbs such as calendula) applied to the scalp can reduce the severity of cradle cap, as long as it is thoroughly rinsed off. Otherwise, the application of oil may actually worsen the problem.

Witch hazel extract, such as that commonly found in the pharmaceutical aisle of the grocery store offers astringent properties that help to reduce the secretions.

Other treatments include simply washing the scalp with a mild, baby friendly shampoo and combing through the affected area to remove the scales.

Cuts / Wounds

What is it? Cuts and scrapes are par for the course for any parent of small children, or anyone that has ever been a small child for that matter. As we go about our daily lives, brushing against or falling over something is bound to happen…more than once.

As long as these cuts are minor, they can be easily treated at home with natural remedies. If the bleeding does not stop or the cut is a large one, a physician should be consulted for treatment, usually stitches or glue.

Likewise, as long as the scrapes and wounds are healing well, they can remain under the care of the home clinic. Should they begin to ooze fluid or become more red and painful after a few days, that is a probable sign of an infection and a trip to the family physician is in order.

Prevention: Caution can prevent many injuries, but considering that cuts and scrapes are rarely intentional, there is not much in the way of prevention that we can do.

Treatments: The first step is to apply direct pressure until the bleeding stops. One the bleeding stops, the goal is to provide clear air for healing, yet keep the affected area clear of germs to prevent an infection. This is much more complicated than it sounds!

Echinacea helps to speed wound healing, while offering antiseptic properties that prevent infection. It is well suited to deeper wounds that need to heal from the inside out, instead of closing quickly, which could lead to infection. Extracts of the herb can be applied topically directly on the scrape or a healing balm can be applied. Personally, I prefer a balm or salve with the herb. Tinctures may sting because of the strong alcohol content, and glycerites are sticky, which would attract dirt. The herb is also suitable for internal use, to help boost the body's own healing process.

Likewise, tea tree oil offers antiseptic properties, which prevent infection. The oil is not suitable for undiluted application on children, but can be mixed with equal parts of olive oil to make a soothing oil.

Calendula, recognized for its anti-inflammatory properties, also promotes wound healing, so when applied topically in a salve or oil, it helps to both reduce inflammation associated with the wound and speed the healing process along.

Dandruff

What is it? Dandruff is an inflammation of the skin, usually occurring on the head that produces embarrassing flakes. Experts disagree on the cause, but potential causes include fungal infections, heredity, or even allergies, and possibly even allergies to the fungus. Other causes of flaky scalp can include cradle cap, contact dermatitis, psoriasis, and a condition known as suborrheic dermatitis.

Prevention: The nutrient biotin is known to help prevent dandruff, so consuming foods rich in biotin such as soy, garlic, avocado, alfalfa, oats and barley is a great preventative measure.

Treatments: Evening primrose oil contains gamma-linolenic acid (GLA), which is converted by the body to anti-inflammatory prostaglandins, which can help with many types of skin rash. Evening primrose is typically sold in a capsule for oral intake, but the capsules can also be broken open and applied directly to the scalp. Other beneficial oils that offer similar properties include flaxseed and fish oil.

Comfrey and plantain both contain allantoin, which is useful at breaking down dandruff scales on the scalp. It is often used for assorted skin disorders to promote wound healing, stimulate cell proliferation and the rebuilding of tissue. Extracts of the herb(s) can be added to commercial natural shampoos. For one application, 5-10 drops of either herb or a blend of the two per tablespoon of shampoo is ideal.

Other beneficial herbs include sage, thyme and rosemary. They can also be added to a shampoo in the above ratio, but are best used in the following hair rinse.

Herbal Hair Rinse
This is a classic old-time herbalists' dandruff treatment, and it has stood the test of time for good reason. While the specific herbs might change based on regional availability or the herbalist's preference, the ingredients generally offer the same basic properties and help to balance the oil production in the scalp, as well as provide protective antiseptic and antifungal properties.

2 cups apple cider vinegar
1 large palmful dried sage, rosemary and thyme
Place the vinegar and herbs into a glass jar; shake well. Store jar in a sunny, warm area and shake it well whenever you pass by. After 10-14 days, strain the herbs. Warm 1/4 cup of the vinegar extract and massage into the scalp. Rinse and repeat daily after shampooing.

Depression

What is it? Clinical depression is not the same as general mood swings that occur in everyday life and should be diagnosed by a professional. Symptoms generally include a series of difficulties in every day life. For examples, both poor appetite and increased appetite can be a sign of depression. Likewise, both insomnia and excessive sleep habits are symptoms, as are both hyperactivity and inactivity.

Considering these wide variances, it is easily understandable that every individual with clinical depression will need a personalized treatment plan. However, there are many similarities that allow us to narrow the choices quite a bit.

Prevention: There are many substances and lifestyle decisions that can contribute to the symptoms of depression. These include alcohol, smoking, lack of exercise and poor diet.

Additionally, some studies show that a diet high in carbohydrates can relieve the symptoms of depression. Of course, we would want to make these healthy carbohydrate choices, as excessive sugars and refined grains can actually trigger some of the same symptoms.

Finally, someone with the symptoms of depression might benefit from checking for underlying disorders. Thyroid problems, hypoglycemia and hormonal imbalances can all lead to symptoms of depression.

Treatments: St. John's wort is the legendary herbal antidepressant. Many clinical studies show that it is more effective at treating clinical depression than pharmaceutical antidepressants (which actually can provide less benefit than a placebo, according to some trials). Long term intake of the herb can lead to an increase sensitivity to sun exposure, so additional sun block may be in order for those that choose to supplement with the herb long term.

Rosemary essential oil helps to stimulate the CNS (Central Nervous System) and can easily be diffused throughout the home or added to cleaning products for double benefits.

Gingko helps to increase the blood flow to the brain, which has been beneficial for many with depression. Gingko also helps the body react to stress, which can worsen or mimic some of the symptoms of depression.

Many individuals with clinical depression have been found to be deficient in assorted B vitamins, especially B6 and folic acid. These vitamins help to keep neurotransmitters high, allowing nerve cells to function normally. Our modern junk food diets and many medications (such as birth control pills) can lead to a deficiency in B vitamins, and depression is a key symptom of a deficiency.

Finally, depression has been linked to food allergies and sensitivities for over 75 years. In 1930, Dr. Albert Rowe, who was one of the leading allergists of the century, coined the term "allergic toxemia" to describe a syndrome that included many of the symptoms of depression. The term is no longer used, but individuals suffering from these symptoms may benefit from food sensitivity testing or an elimination diet.

Detoxification

What is it? Detoxification is not an illness, rather a term given to the act of intentionally aiding the body in its natural process of riding itself of toxins. The process to a lesser extent is ongoing, thanks to the fervent work of our liver and naturally designed cleansing functions, but sometimes, especially in our polluted environment, additional help can bring about health benefits.

Treatments: There are many different types of detoxification that an individual can choose to use. Some of them are simple and mild, while others can be quite strong and even harsh. Choosing which type of detox to take can often be a difficult challenge.

Studies show that organic fruits and vegetables have far more antioxidants than the conventional version. This varies based on the food tested and the study, but some studies show as many as ten times the antioxidants in organic foods. Additionally, many foods have been found to contain significantly more antioxidants than others. Foods especially rich in antioxidants include: berries (the darker the better), broccoli, tomatoes, spinach, carrots, whole grains, artichokes, beans, apples and pecans. Tea, especially green tea is also rich in antioxidants. Research also shows that the majority of the antioxidant rich foods fall under the herb and spice category. By adding a dash of this and a sprinkle of that, not only do we add flavor to our meals, we also add important health benefits.

Liver support, in the form of milk thistle or dandelion, also helps assist the body in its natural detoxification system. These herbs can be obtained in liquid extract or in capsules, often with mild laxatives such as oats or flax added to help along the elimination process. Milk thistle should be standardized to contain at least 80% silymarin, which is the active set of compounds.

Diabetes

What is it? When the body has a difficult time regulating its blood sugar levels or blood glucose, we term the condition diabetes. There are two main types, type 1 and type 2.

Type 1 was previously called juvenile diabetes or insulin dependent diabetes and is a disorder of the body's immune system. When the pancreas is attacked and beta cells are destroyed, insulin production is hindered. Without insulin, sugar in the body is not processed as normal, and is left to damage major organs in the body, while the cells are not receiving the energy they need. Many researchers believe that exposure in infancy to bovine alumni peptide, a protein in cow's milk, can lead to the autoimmune process that leads to type 1 diabetes.

However, less that 10% of individuals with diabetes suffer from type 1. Over 90% are diagnosed with type 2 diabetes, which is when insulin is not sufficiently produced and / or the body is not properly using the insulin. This type is linked to dietary and lifestyle choices.

Prevention: Once again, a whole foods diet and active lifestyle is the key to prevention. Diabetes is not often found in cultures that consume a traditional, natural diet, yet is a common sight in more "modern" societies. However, as these cultures begin to change to our modern diets, the occurrence begins to closely match our own.

Obesity is another major factor in type two diabetes, so maintaining a healthy weight (again through a whole foods diet and active lifestyle) is a great preventative measure, especially for those with a family history of insulin resistance.

Prevention for children can also begin prior to their birth. Research shows that children born to mothers that carefully controlled their blood sugar during pregnancy through healthy dietary choices are 50% less likely to experience type two diabetes. Controlling blood sugar is not the same as dieting or restricting caloric intake during pregnancy, rather it refers to choosing healthy carbohydrate, protein and fat options during this critical time in the child's development.

Treatments: Both types of diabetes are within the scope of natural medicine, however type one diabetes should not be treated at home without the assistance of a licensed physician properly trained in natural medicine.

Chromium is the active component of the body's glucose tolerance factor, which increases the action of insulin. It is believed to initiate the attachment of insulin to insulin receptors. It cannot be combined with insulin medication since it can actually cause blood sugar levels to drop, so it is best used for moderate treatment of individuals that are not taking insulin regularly. Certain foods are naturally rich in chromium, including onions, romaine lettuce, tomatoes, whole grains and potatoes (surprisingly). Supplementation is best when taken in a chelated form with picolinate, and should not be combined with pain relievers such as ibuprofen, naproxen or aspirin.

Fenugreek contains compounds that help to regulate blood sugar levels, making it ideal for those with prediabetes, especially when obesity or poor diet are factors.

Gynmena is historic botanical treatment for blood sugar problems, It decreases the caloric intake during a meal and helps to enhance glucose control. It is suspected that this is caused by an increase in insulin production. Studies also seem to support the idea that gynmena can actually regenerate the pancreatic cells in humans with both types of diabetes.

Bay leaves also help the body to use insulin more effectively, which can be beneficial for those with prediabetes or mild diabetes. As a culinary herb, bay leaves can be added liberally to the diet to take advantage of these benefits.

The traditional diabetes diet includes an abundance of protein, which is digested more slowly than carbohydrates, combined with a reduction of carbohydrate consumption. This helps to avoid the blood sugar spikes and resulting "lows" that often occur. However, another approach has recently been studied with great success. When compared to the traditional diabetes diet, a vegan diet was shown in one trial to increase weight loss and reverse diabetes, controlling blood sugar levels three times better. This research may lead to a new path in the dietary treatment of both types of diabetes.

Diarrhea

What is it? Diarrhea is characterized by sudden loose stools, with an increased frequency. It is often accompanied by cramping and can lead to dehydration. Common causes of diarrhea include food poisoning, food allergies or sensitivities, antibiotics and other medications. Any diarrhea that is severe or persists longer than 3 days without any sign of relief should be evaluated by the family physician to rule out underlying causes or possible dehydration.

Prevention: Many causes of diarrhea can be prevented by simply increasing our awareness and adaptation of healthy habits. Hand washing, especially after trips to the restroom greatly diminishes the occurrence of diarrhea, since many of the causes of diarrhea are directly linked to proper hygienic practices.

Responsible use of antibiotics can also decrease the occurrence of diarrhea, and when antibiotics are genuinely warranted, supplementation with a good quality probiotic blend can decrease the potential for diarrhea.

For children with chronic diarrhea, the cause is often a simple milk intolerance or sensitivity. Experts project that the actual number of individuals that cannot tolerate milk is much higher than we all realize.

Young children and toddlers are especially prone, as their digestive tracts are not often mature enough to digest these proteins properly. This can be avoided or corrected by simply switching over to nutritionally superior goat's milk. It contains greater amounts of naturally homogenized fat, many more essential fatty acids, more calcium, Vitamin B6, Vitamin A, potassium, niacin, copper and selenium. Furthermore, the proteins in goat milk are much more similar to the proteins in breastmilk, which makes them better suited for the young digestive tract.

Treatments: The first line of treatment with diarrhea is to watch carefully for dehydration. Common electrolyte drinks often contain artificial sugars, food dyes and artificial flavors, none of which should be given to children, especially not sick children. Instead, I opt for a natural electrolyte drink from a health food store or a homemade version.

Herbal teas also help to increase the fluid intake and bring about relief. Blackberry and raspberry leaves, as well as common black tea leaves all offer astringent properties that help treat the diarrhea.

Probiotic blends are always indicated in the case of intestinal troubles. Age specific blends from a reputable source are going to provide maximum benefit.

Carob powder is also a reliable treatment and in one trial sped up the healing process so much that it decreased the duration of the diarrhea from 4 days to an average of 2 days. Carob powder can be combined with applesauce and cinnamon for added benefits such as tannins, pectin and astringent properties, all of which bring about a speedier recovery. The applesauce should be natural or homemade, however, to avoid any laxative properties found in the juice!

Homemade Electrolyte Drinks:
1 cup purified water
1/3 cup grape juice / orange juice / berry juice (organic)
1/4 teaspoon pure mineral salt
Pinch baking soda
Blend all ingredients well and serve chilled.

Diaper Rash

What is it? Diaper rash is a catchall term for any rash that occurs in the diaper area. These rashes can result in reddish, tender skin or the flaming bright red lesions that cause great pain. While they were once referred to as ammonia burns, diaper rashes now are due to an assortment of factors. Some of the most common types of diaper rash are yeast rashes, allergic reaction rashes, rashes from diarrhea, impetigo, and the classic ammonia rash.

Prevention: The best way to prevent diaper rash is to keep the baby's bum dry and clean. Properly changing diapers when they are wet or soiled will ensure the bum is exposed to the fewest number of irritants. (A baby should go no longer than 2-3 hours during the day between changes, whether or not the diaper has reached its peak capacity.) Cloth diapers are a good option for babies with sensitive skin. Another prevention measure is to allow for "free time" when the bum is diaper free. If a mom is undertaking elimination communication or natural infant hygiene, this is accomplished much easier.

Other prevention measures include checking closely for food allergies and applying a protective balm to the bum during bouts of diarrhea or illness.

Treatments: Once a rash occurs, the first step in treatment is to ensure it does not get any worse. This can be done by applying pure olive oil or an anti-inflammatory salve to the area creating a barrier between the diaper and bum, which protects the bottom from the eliminated waste.

To treat the actual rash, balms and salves are ideal, since they can actually seal in the area, offering both protection and treatment at the same time. Herbs to include in a homemade balm include echinacea, chamomile, calendula, plantain and lavender. After the salve is cooled, tea tree oil can be added for further benefit.

If natural diapering solutions such as cloth diapers or natural infant hygiene are not feasible, natural wipe solutions can be used instead of or in addition to conventional wipes. These are ideal for sensitive skin, and can be preventative in nature as well. My favorite wipe solution formula is below.

Baby Bum Wipes
In a large glass mixing bowl, combine 1 1/2 cups witch hazel extract with 1/4 cup vegetable glycerin and 3T olive oil. Mix well. Add 1 t calendula extract, 6 drops lavender oil and 3 drops tea tree oil. Pour into a sterile bottle. This can be used with a spray top and sprayed onto each wipe prior to use, but I prefer to use a plain cap and pour some out onto the cloth wipes to ensure the wipe is thoroughly moistened. The mixture will often separate as it sits, so be sure to shake well before opening.

Diverticulitis

What is it? Diverticulitis is the term given to the condition in which the diverticula, which are small balloon-like protrusions in the intestinal wall, become inflamed or infected. While the pockets are common in individuals over the age of forty, the infection and inflammation occurs as a result of a low fiber diet or a weakness in the intestinal wall. Without the inflammation, there are generally no symptoms caused by the balloon-like diverticula, although they do remain in the colon for life.

Symptoms of diverticulitis infections include fever, nausea, vomiting, rectal bleeding, bloating and abdominal pain in the lower left side. Much like appendicitis, if severe diverticulitis remains untreated, the infection can cause a rupture, which is always a medical emergency.

Prevention: Constipation is a contributing factor in diverticulitis, and it is much more common in countries such as the United States, where individuals tend to consume a low fiber diet. Stress is another trigger, and when combined with poor diet places an individual at high risk for developing diverticula, which can easily become scraped, often resulting in inflammation and infection.

Therefore, prevention of diverticulitis revolves around consuming a healthy, whole foods diet rich in plant fibers and low in animal products.

This is a classic example of how our diet affects us more profoundly as we age, and how important a role prevention and nutrition actually play in our overall health.

Treatment: Considering that the main cause of diverticulitis is a low fiber diet, the best way to treat diverticulitis is to include more fiber in the diet. Psyllium husks help ensure that the bowels are thoroughly emptied as they should be, and that constipation does not occur. Psyllium is easy to find in health food snack bars or as a powder to toss onto a salad. Generally, up to 1 teaspoon of the husks are sufficient for an entire day. They can also be purchased in pill form, but it may take 4-6 pills to get the same amount of benefit, as bulk fiber cannot be concentrated.

Probiotics are always an important supplement to consider when intestinal problems are present. As waste sits in the bowels, it can putrify, causing bacterial overgrowth and other health concerns. Probiotics help to correct this imbalance, and prevent it from occurring again.

Peppermint is an effective digestive aid, alleviates inflammation and ensures a healthy balance of intestinal flora. It also contains antispasmodic properties that prevent the cramping and discomfort. One to two enteric coated capsules ensure that the potent oil makes it through the digestive juices for maximum absorption. This can be taken 2-3 times a day.

Garlic helps to ensure that the intestinal flora is in the correct ratios, and fights off bacterial infections in the intestines. Kyolic odorless capsules are a great product to obtain these benefits for intestinal trouble.

Slippery elm bark provides mucilagenous properties that actually soothe the inflamed intestines, providing quick relief. It also functions as a mild laxative, keeping things moving right along, thereby preventing the intense outbreaks.

Chamomile is another great treatment for the condition. Not only does chamomile help to alleviate stress, which is a known contributing factor to outbreaks, it also functions as a digestive aid, ensuring our food makes its way successfully all the way through our system, instead of stopping along the way, and it contains powerful anti-inflammatory actions that soothe the inflamed intestines.

Ear Infection

What is it? According to the National Institute of Health, ear infections are the most common illness among babies and children. They are most often found in the middle ear, which is termed otitis media, and they usually go away on their own, requiring no further treatment than comfort measures and pain relief. Yet, an estimated 5 billion (yes, billion) dollars are spent annually on medical costs and lost wages. Seventy five percent of children have at least one infection by the age of 3 and almost half of them have 3 or more by that age.

The treatment of ear infections is by far one of the most controversial topics in the pediatric world today. I find this highly unfortunate, as the treatment guidelines are actually very clear. The controversy appears to stem from care providers and parents that have deep seated notions that are not quite up to par with modern research and evidenced based medicine.

The American Academy of Pediatrics has been issuing statements since 1997 against the routine use of antibiotics for ear infections. The reasoning for this is two fold. First, research has not shown antibiotic treatment to shorten the duration of the infection. Second, the routine use of antibiotics when not warranted, such as a routine ear infection, leads to antibiotic resistance bacteria, which according to the World Health Organization, is one of the most pressing issues of our day.

Prevention: Generally speaking, ear infections follow a cold or flu when fluids have had a chance to pool in the inner ear. Once these accumulated fluids remain stagnant, the tendency to become infected is pretty high. To compound the problem, antibiotic use, which is actually still common among some care providers, dramatically increases the rate of recurring infections, each one becoming more and more difficult to treat.

Therefore, our best prevention measure is to prevent the fluid from pooling in the ear, or assist its drainage if it does occur. One great way to do this is to elevate the head during a cold and to take measures to boost the immune system.

Additionally, studies suggest that milk allergies and sensitivities often present themselves in the form of ear infections. Often times, the simple act of eliminating dairy from the diet will resolve the problem.

Treatments: Since we know that many ear infections will resolve themselves without our assistance, our first treatment measure is to provide some comfort and pain relief for the child. The best herbs for this are calendula and mullein. Both of these herbs are anti-inflammatory, which helps to soothe the irritated membranes and alleviate some of the inflammation.

To combat infection, garlic oil is the first line of defense among most herbalists. This oil is antibacterial, and when applied directly into the ear (via a carrier oil), is highly effective.

For another treatment option, an herbal blend of calendula, garlic, mullein, chamomile and lavender has actually been shown to decrease the duration of the infection, providing both immediate relief and infection fighting properties. Herbs for Kids produces a blend for ear infections with many of the same properties as the herbs mentioned above, and is readily available at most health food stores.

Finally, as mentioned above, the root cause of the infection is the accumulation of fluid pooling in the ear. While we rid ourselves of the infection, we must also consider the removal of the fluid to be paramount to recovery. This may seem like an insurmountable task, but there are many simple massage options that are quite effective. One option that I highly recommend is found in the book *No More Amoxicillin* by Dr. Mary Anne Block. She is an osteopathic physician and the technique is an osteopathic one that is highly effective. I cannot recommend her book enough.

I also often use a basic massage technique in my own home for quick relief:

First, lay the child on his back. In a circular motion, massage the lymph nodes on the upper chest to stimulate them. Next, gently stroke the sides of the face, one at a time. Begin at the side of the face in front of the ears. Using a small amount of firm pressure, gently move downwards to the jaw line and follow towards the front of the face. Repeat 2-3 times per side. As an additional relaxation measure (though unnecessary for the ear drainage), while the child is being massaged, you can place both thumbs at the inner point of the eyebrows. Gently, but firmly rub towards the outside to the hairline. An herbal massage oil with a bit of eucalyptus added can be used to assist in clear breathing and relaxation during a cold. (No more than 1 drop of essential oil per 2-3 tablespoons of carrier oil.)

Eczema

What is it? While the official name for eczema is atopic dermatitis, the word has become a catch all term for all forms of skin dermatitis, which affect an estimated 1 in 3 individuals. Many types of dermatitis actually exist, however, and each has its own causes and treatments, which is why natural "cures" for eczema can be so varied.

Common complaints include overall dry skin, patches of especially dry and flaky skin and the dreaded "flare up" which results in itchy, extremely dry and sometimes cracked and bleeding patches on the skin.

Eczema has often been considered to be an allergic disorder, but recent research also indicates that genetics are strongly involved.

It is important to remember that eczema is not the problem; it is a compilation of symptoms of an underlying problem (such as an allergy) and is our body's way of letting us know something is wrong. So, our prevention and treatment in a natural setting will reflect this concept by focusing not on the symptoms of eczema, but the underlying cause or the source of the main problem.

Prevention: Considering the underlying causes, prevention focuses on reducing or eliminating potential triggers or determining factors of the irritation. This includes the removal of possible skin irritants, including soaps, body care products, laundry soaps, certain clothing material, and even airborne household toxins. Certainly I am not suggesting that we live our lives free from soap and skin care, rather these items should be removed and replaced with a natural version that can provide benefits to the skin. Instead of soap, a natural soap free skin cleanser should be used, followed by organic or truly natural skin care products, which can be made at home using some of the formulas in the back of this book or purchased at a health food store. The same applies to our laundry soaps, air fresheners, and other household items. Quite honestly, the natural versions are much more luxurious, so this is a trade off with multiple perks!

Dietary allergies or sensitivities can be determined by obtaining food sensitivity testing through a naturally minded physician or by undertaking an elimination diet. This is accomplished by removing questionable offenders from the diet for a period of time (often 3-4 weeks) and then testing the food by consuming again. If it is causing problems, the symptoms should decrease during the avoidance period, but reappear within a few days of the challenge test.

Treatments: The first line of defense in my practice is to discuss milk thistle supplementation. Milk thistle is a liver supportive herb. Since our liver is our detoxification organ, this can help assist with the efficient removal of toxins from the body and reduce the skin irritation. Many wellness experts believe that the skin is a great indicator as to the health of the liver. Milk thistle is a gentle herb and one that is used daily in many countries for boosting the natural detoxification process through the liver.

The herbs burdock and dandelion also help relieve eczema when applied topically. The best way to achieve this is to place the dried herbs into a tea bag and steep in warm water. The moist bags are placed onto the affected areas (but not broken skin) and the potent water can also be applied directly for 5-10 minutes. Once the treatment is complete, the skin can be sealed with a natural moisturizer, locking in the valuable properties.

Comfrey and licorice creams also offer great benefit, comparable to that of traditional cortisone creams. These can be found at a health food store or made at home by adding 4-6 drops of each in extract form to a couple of tablespoons of a natural skin moisturizer directly before application.

The improper metabolism of fatty acids is also a common culprit. This can be addressed by supplementing with zinc, which is essential for the metabolism process and by adding additional omega 3 fatty acids to the diet. Not only are these generally lacking in individuals with eczema, they offer anti-inflammatory properties, which benefit the skin through topical application as well. The most common and easy to find sources include fish oil, flax oil and evening primrose oil.

Endometriosis

What is it? In roughly 3%-5% of the female population, tissue resembling the uterine lining (the endometrium) begins to grow outside of the uterus in the ovaries, fallopian tubes, cervix, bowel or bladder. Once this tissue begins to grow there, it swells and bleeds along with the monthly cycle, causing pain, excessive bleeding, cramping, irregular periods and even infertility. It can also cause intercourse to be painful.

This problem generally makes itself known between the ages of 25 and 40, but experts do not know when it actually begins. They also do not know what causes it and there is not a reliable treatment for it, although when the estrogen levels are under control, it often becomes inactive, with no symptoms.

Prevention: While there is no generally accepted evidence of what causes endometriosis, there is one prevailing theory that has some good preliminary evidence behind it, so it is worth consideration. Evidence seems to suggest that the immune system becomes damaged by estrogen-like environmental pollutants, including pesticides. Other culprits are immune suppressing drugs and dietary toxins. Avoidance of these substances can bring about other health benefits as well, so it is certainly worth trying.

Treatments: One of the primary treatments for estrogen-related problems is the use of phytoestrogens. These plant estrogens can actually adhere to the receptor sites in the body, preventing the storage of estrogen, and actually blocking estrogen in the body.

Cramp bark has been used successfully for many years to relax the uterine muscles, treating menstrual cramps, easing childbirth and preventing miscarriage. This herb would offer similar benefits during a painful experience with endometriosis. Women that do not have kidney stones can take up to three cups of tea a day. Women with kidney stones should avoid cramp bark.

Yarrow helps to reduce cramps and inflammation, as well as slow excessive bleeding, which is common with endometriosis. For a standard 1:5 tincture, 3/4 teaspoon can be taken 3 times per day, beginning 7-10 days before a period, and ending 10-14 days afterwards.

Red raspberry is a favorite among midwives for strengthening the uterus, preparing it for childbirth, but this can also benefit women with endometriosis, as it can also help relieve heavy periods. The tea acts as an astringent on the body, and is safe enough to take up to 8 or even 10 cups a day.

Considering that research shows us that when the estrogen levels are dropped, the symptoms disappear, I would also suggest milk thistle for anyone with endometriosis. Boosting the liver's function will help to eliminate excess hormones from the body more efficiently, which may bring about this cease in symptoms.

Excitability

What is it? All of us tend to get excited about holidays, vacations, and other fun activities, but when children are excited about something, they tend to allow the excitement to overshadow their behavioral guidelines and their need for sleep. This can lead to further health concerns, and even a decreased immune response.

Prevention: Life is full of fun and memorable events, and there is really no way to prevent these things from happening. Why would we want to?

Treatments: When the excitement of the day's events (or the anticipation of the day's events) becomes so great that it interferes with behavioral guidelines or sleep habits, we can turn to some gentle herbs to alleviate the excess of energy.

Chamomile is the perfect herb for calming and soothing an overly excited child. Peter Rabbit's mother had it right all along, as she gave the little bunny some chamomile tea to relax him for bed after a day full of excitement. Our children may not be bunnies, but they do benefit from this use of the herb.

Bach Rescue Remedy is one of the Bach flower remedies that is designed to calm intense emotions and is perfectly suitable for helping little ones gain some control during an eventful day. The dose should be adjusted to account for their smaller size.

If it is bedtime and the excitement is too much to bear, some of the herbs listed under insomnia may be beneficial, but it is important to remember that these sedatives should only be taken if the individual is ready for bed and has enough time to get a good night's sleep. Otherwise, the sleepy child (or parent) combined with a day of excitement can be a recipe for disaster!

Eyesight, poor

What is it? Eyesight is something we often take for granted, especially if we are some of the few that don't require any assistance at any time to go about our daily activities. For those that do, however, poor eyesight rarely leaves their minds for too long.

While there is no herbal cure that brings eyesight back to 20/20, there are substances that can help to halt the eyesight from getting worse, and some are even thought to bring about some relief.

Prevention: For the most part, eyesight changes without much action on our part, however, consuming a healthy diet rich in antioxidants helps to ensure that the body has all it needs to prevent it from getting worse.

Additionally, most specialists agree that regular check ups and contacts or glasses that are the correct prescription for the individual help prevent eyesight damage that comes from neglect. So, if you wear contacts, don't delay getting that check up and new lenses annually!

Treatments: Bilberry, a relative of blueberry, can strengthen the capillaries of the eye, preventing the bloodshot appearance of strained eyes, and boosting the vision potential. It also helps to improve night vision and increase the visual field, according to researchers. While bilberry seems to be the one in the spotlight, the active compounds in the fruit are also in blueberries, cranberries and grapes, so the inclusion of these foods into the diet is very beneficial for those with eye problems.

Fatigue

What is it? As I write this, it is well past midnight, and I already know how that is going to affect me tomorrow. Only, fatigue like I will feel is understandable. It is my body telling me I should have gotten more sleep! Sometimes, however, fatigue is not directly related to staying up late to finish a project or tending to a sick or teething child. Sometimes fatigue just affects us for what seems to be no reason at all.

Of course, there is a reason, even though we have not found it. Fatigue is often a result of a nutritional deficiency. Iron deficient anemia is a common cause. Thyroid problems, sleep disorders and pharmaceutical drugs are other causes.

In the absence of an underlying cause, fatigue is usually the result of our lifestyles stressing out our bodies too much. Our habits of staying up too late, rising too early and running from dawn to dusk cannot be continued without affecting the body somehow, and fatigue is a common result.

Prevention: Since fatigue is often caused by our stressful lifestyles, the best prevention is to take a break from time to time and allow the body to catch up with us! Taking a rest day each week to relax and enjoy what we have been blessed with helps to bring about emotional and physical health.

Treatments: Adaptogens, one of my favorite classifications of herbs, are well suited to treat fatigue. Astragalus root helps the body respond to stress and increases the white blood count, boosting the immune system, which is notoriously low when experiencing fatigue.

Rosemary essential oil also helps to stimulate the central nervous system, improving memory and enhancing cognitive function in general. It is best used by dilution throughout a room, 1-2 drops at a time.

Another common and very natural stimulant, caffeine, is effective at boosting the energy levels, but should not be considered a long term solution. While it is certainly beneficial (for those that do not have hypertension), prolonged use can over stimulate the adrenal glands, which can actually cause fatigue.

Fever

What is it? A fever is a sign that the body is fighting off something. Contrary to popular thought, fevers are not usually a concern, as they are a beneficial part of our natural disease fighting process.

Occasionally, certain fevers are signs of something that requires immediate medical attention. A fever should be considered a cause for concern if any of the following are present:

> A baby younger than 3 months has a fever higher than 100.4
> An older child has a fever higher than 104
> A high fever cannot be brought down
> Any other signs are combined with the fever, including stiff neck, persistent and inconsolable crying, lethargy (not a tired baby, but truly lethargic), difficulty breathing or signs of dehydration

Contacting outside help for these concerns is not usually something mothers enjoy, as the additional diagnostic measures are often very uncomfortable, but these measures are necessary as the symptoms can reflect serious and fast acting diseases. Our personal experience is that our local hospital and family physician always begin with the least invasive procedures and try to avoid progressing to more invasive procedures unless absolutely necessary.

Prevention: Considering that the fever is a sign of an illness, not an illness itself, there is no specific prevention measure for fever.

Treatments: Fevers are vital parts to the disease fighting system of our fearfully and wonderfully made bodies. Therefore, as long as the fever is mild, we generally do not treat it, instead allowing the fever to work. The increased heat is uncomfortable for us, but works to kill viruses and other illness in the body. Reducing the mild fever inhibits the body's natural line of defense against the illness, leaving us more susceptible to harm. If the fever is mild enough that we are not treating it, we remain vigilant to observe it, ensuring it remains under control, and we supplement with added fluids to remain hydrated.

When a fever rises beyond the "mild" classification to moderate or high, it is time to consider treatment. In the Hawkins' home, the magical number is 103, but each house should, with input from the family physician, determine what number they are comfortable with. One of our first actions is a mild, moderately warm bath. Cool baths can cause shivering, which can then increase the temperature, but a milder bath can help lower the temperature without causing the chills.

We also use a blend called Children's Composition, which is available from many different brands. Herbs for Kids brand labels their blend Temp Assure. This blend helps boost immune function and can keep a temperature under control. These blends include peppermint, echinacea, elder and yarrow.

If we do find ourselves treating a higher fever with an over the counter supplement, such as acetaminophen, we should be careful to always include milk thistle supplementation to protect the liver from possible harm.

Food Sensitivity

What is it? A food sensitivity is a reaction to a food that causes unwanted and often harmful effects on the body, but is not a food allergy. Food sensitivities are very common, although many individuals do not even realize that they have a sensitivity unless the effects are dramatic.

Prevention: The exact cause of a sensitivity is unclear, but when a food is consumed too often, and there is damage to the intestinal walls leading to increased gut permeability, the constant exposure to a particular food can then trigger a reaction. Ensuring that the diet has plenty of variety and a healthy intestinal flora can help prevent this from happening.

Treatments: Since food sensitivities are not true allergies, they can usually be treated and reversed somewhat quickly. The basic plan is to first determine which food are causing the problems. An elimination diet is a great tool, or a physician can run a blood test (called the ELISA) to determine which foods are causing reactions.

To do an elimination diet, first choose foods that are potential reactors. Often, this will be the foods most often craved. Remove them from the diet for 3-4 weeks as a trial period. The symptoms should disappear during this time, or at least be less severe. Then, to challenge the food, consume it liberally for a day. If symptoms reappear, the food is a culprit. Offensive foods often have what is called a delayed reaction, not showing any symptoms for a few days. If symptoms do not change after a week, the food is fine.

Once these foods are removed from the diet, supplementation with probiotics, digestive enzymes and fish or flax oil are taken while the body has a chance to heal. After 4-6 months, the food can be reintroduced again as another challenge test. Eventually the food can be brought back into the diet without reactions.

Gallstones

What is it? The gallbladder is a small sac of fluid that holds bile, which helps our body to properly digest fats. When cholesterol or even calcium becomes concentrated in the gallbladder, they can crystallize, forming hard lumps that can range from the size of a grain of salt to larger than a golf ball.

Gallstones are more common in women than men, and part of this is a direct result of childbearing. During pregnancy, the cholesterol in the body increases substantially, and the balance of cholesterol and bile is altered. This leads to an increase in gallbladder attacks during pregnancy or in the postpartum period.

Most of the time, these stones are harmless and painless. However, if one of the stones begins to block one of the ducts leading from the gallbladder to the liver or small intestines, serious problems can occur, and we call this a gallbladder attack.

Such attacks can cause severe pain, most notably in the upper right abdomen, fever, nausea, and even vomiting. These symptoms can last from a couple of minutes to a few hours.

Traditional allopathic care includes the removal of the gallbladder, but natural health experts argue that the removal of an organ rarely contributes to an improvement of overall health. I certainly wouldn't drive my car if parts have been removed, and our bodies are a much more intricate and complex creation than our vehicles.

Prevention: The ideal form of prevention for gallstones includes consuming a near vegetarian diet, low in cholesterol and rich in fiber and antioxidants. This prevents the opportunity for cholesterol to become over saturated, forming stones.

Abundant consumption of fat, protein, and sugar also make an individual more prone to gallstones, and high cholesterol plays an obvious role.

Treatments: Our lowly thistles play a major role in the treatment of gallstones. Artichokes help the body to digest fats properly and can actually lower cholesterol. The best way to take advantage of these benefits is to add the food, not a supplement, to the diet on a regular basis.

Milk thistle assists the liver's functioning, and also increases bile solubility. This helps to dissolve and eliminate stones and prevent the recurrence. Dandelion, another liver boosting herb helps to promote bile production. Increased bile production is beneficial because it reduces the chance for the cholesterol to become oversaturated.

Herbs in the mint family, especially peppermint, also help to dissolve gallstones and prevent them from blocking the ducts. Peppermint tea is a great treatment method, but enteric coated capsules of the essential oil taken 2 times a day between meals can ensure the benefits make it through the digestive fluids.

GERD

What is it? Gastrointestinal Esophageal Reflux Disorder, commonly called reflux, is a term to define the spilling out of partially digested food and hydrochloric acid from the stomach back up into the esophagus. While the stomach is lined with protective mucus to prevent damage from the extremely low pH of our stomach acid, the rest of our delicate tissues are left unprotected and can be easily damaged by such a strong acid.

The lower esophageal sphincter (LES) is a round muscle that opens to allow the passage of food into the stomach, but then closes, keeping the contents down. When it is weakened, it can easily reopen, allowing the contents to slip back up.

Reflux is a disorder that conventional (or allopathic) medicine and natural medicine greatly disagree on. Allopathic medicine assures us that reflux is caused by too much stomach acid, and that we should work to reduce, suppress or neutralize the acid in the stomach.

Yet, there is substantial evidence to support the viewpoint that there is actually not an abundance of hydrochloric acid, rather a deficiency of hydrochloric acid in individuals with reflux, which would mean that our standard treatments are actually prolonging the problem, which may be the reason we seldom observe an individual recover from reflux with our conventional treatments. One physician in private practice found that over 90% of his patients with reflux showed insufficient levels of hydrochloric acid, when tested.

Prevention: Numerous lifestyle habits can lead to GERD, including overeating, eating too quickly and emotional stress or nervousness during mealtime. NSAIDS can also lead to reflux. These include over the counter remedies such as ibuprofen, aspirin and naproxen.

Poor dietary and lifestyle choices are also factors, especially fatty and fried foods, sugar, smoking, carbonated beverages and too little water.

Treatments: A first line of treatment from a natural standpoint would be to add plenty of digestive aids to the routine. Peppermint capsules (enteric coated are ideal), ginger tea or extract and chamomile tea all work to improve our digestion, easing the symptoms and preventing the situation from worsening.

Existing burns can be treated with soothing herbs containing plenty of mucilage. Slippery elm bark tablets are easy to find in a health food store in the cold and flu section, as they also make great cough drops.

Licorice is a standard treatment for reflux, but has come under scrutiny lately because of a compound found in the herb. However, studies show that deglycyrrhizinated licorice, which has the harmful compound removed, is just as effective at treating reflux and is safe for general adult use.

Finally, all intestinal problems generally benefit from the addition of probiotics to the routine. These beneficial bacteria strands help to maintain the proper intestinal flora, reducing the numbers of harmful bacteria and yeasts in the intestines and ensuring healthy digestion. This step is critical for those that have routinely taken antacids, as these effectively reduce the acidity of the stomach. The stomach was designed to have a low pH, as this helps to prevent the growth of harmful bacteria, ensuring continual health. When this natural system is disturbed with medication, harmful bacteria are allowed to thrive, causing further complications. Furthermore, these low acid levels in the body are suspected to increase the occurrence of stomach cancers and can inhibit the absorption of essential nutrients.

Hair Loss

What is it? Our bodies naturally lose some hair throughout the day, but this is to be expected and new growth generally replaces all that was lost. When the hair loss begins to exceed the new growth, it leads to overall thinness as the scalp begins to show through.

The most common causes of hair loss come with age and are referred to as male pattern baldness or female pattern baldness. Yes, hair loss actually affects both males and females. Hormonal changes and nutritional deficiencies can also lead to hair loss.

Prevention: A whole foods diet is the best prevention for decreasing the occurrence of hair loss.

Treatments: Gingko helps to improve circulation to the scalp, which can stimulate new hair growth. It also helps to improve cognitive function, which is an added benefit.

Rosemary oil, another memory enhancer, helps to stimulate the growth of new hair. The best way to take advantage of these benefits is to add a single drop to a dollop of shampoo before massaging into the scalp. Massage thoroughly and repeat daily for best results.

Saw palmetto also plays a significant role in battling male hair loss, as it prevents the conversion of the male sex hormone testosterone into dihydrotestosterone, more simply known as DHT. This substance damages the hair follicles, which of course, prevents the growth of new hair. This treatment then helps to slow hair loss, but not reverse it.

Considering that saw palmetto also plays a valuable role in preventing prostate enlargement, it is an ideal supplement for aging males.

Halitosis

What is it? Halitosis is nothing more than the formal name for the dreaded case of bad breath. Having unpleasant breath is normal under certain circumstances, such as a garlic laden pasta for lunch or a day without brushing, but chronic bad breath, especially bad breath that does not seem to go away, despite the best oral hygiene, may be a sign of an underlying problem or infection. Chronic halitosis typically requires a trip to the dentist for further examination.

Prevention: In many cases, bad breath is caused by nothing more than inadequate hydration. Saliva cleanses the mouth, removing oral bacteria and particles of food that may be lingering from the last meal. When we have plenty of saliva, this process helps greatly in keeping our breath fresh smelling.

Treatments: The first line of defense for most bad breath is a simple mouthwash to rinse and cleanse the environment. Yet, most over the counter mouthwashes offer little in terms of prevention or cure. Traditional mouthwashes that are effective include potent herbs that will both rinse the area and thoroughly cleanse it. It is actually quite easy to make your own mouthwash at home, and adjusting the flavor to suit your tastes can be a fun afternoon project!

In addition to mouthwash, traditional breath fresheners included actually chewing potent herbs between and after meals. Herbs such as parsley, mint and tarragon are good ideas. One main ingredient in parsley, chlorophyll, is highly effective at ensuring sweet smelling breath. Since most of us prefer not to chew parsley all day, we can also supplement with pure chlorophyll instead. This can be found in a health food store.

Homemade mouthwash:
Fill a glass canning jar with 2 cups vodka. Add a combination of the following dried herbs to total 1/2 cup: peppermint, spearmint, lavender, basil, sage, tarragon, cinnamon or rosemary. Shake well and allow to sit in a warm sunlit spot for 2-4 weeks, shaking daily. After the infusion is complete, strain out the herbs and pour into a bottle. At this point, you can add 10-15 drops of one of the following optional oils: lemon, lavender, sweet orange or lime. Be sure to label the bottle with the ingredients and date. It is also important to include a warning not to consume the product, since mouthwash is a rinse out product, and we don't want members of our household ingesting the strong product.

Hand Foot Mouth

What is it? This common childhood illness presents itself with a fever, sores in the mouth, and a rash with blisters. Other symptoms include a sore throat, mild fatigue, and decreased appetite. The sores begin as small red spots that develop into blisters. They begin in the mouth but usually spread to the palms of the hands and feet.

This is not the same thing as foot and mouth, which is a common disease of cattle. It is usually caused by coxsackievirus, which is contagious but usually mild and passes quickly among children under the age of ten years. Without treatment, most individuals recover within 7-10 days.

Prevention: Hand foot and mouth disease is prevented by boosting the immune system (a crucial step in natural health), and the avoidance of others with the contagious illness. It is commonly spread among day care centers and preschools, so additional attention should be given to the immune systems of children in those settings.

Treatments: Chamomile tea offers anti-inflammatory properties that help relieve the discomfort in the mouth. For a special treat, freeze the tea in popsicle molds for a frozen treatment.

Immune boosting herbs such as elderberry extract and astragalus root can help the body fight it off faster, and plenty of fluids ensure that discomfort is kept at a minimum.

The hands and feet, if affected, can be placed in herbal soaks made from astringent herbs such as raspberry and blackberry leaves. Calendula flowers can be added to the blend for some anti-inflammatory properties. Simply toss the dried herbs into a warm water bath and let the hands or feet soak as the herbs infuse the water.

Hay fever

What is it? I am reminded of the source of the word "hay fever" every time I spend more than 5 minutes in the barn where my daughter tends to the horses she is learning to ride. I can usually tell you in a matter of seconds whether or not her trainer has had a recent delivery of hay, because my eyes glaze over, then become red and inflamed. This is quickly followed by intense sneezing and a nonstop "runny nose", and any individual that has experienced hay fever, more commonly referred to as allergies, can attest to the misery that follows.

Prevention: Insufficient hydration can make an individual more prone to hay fever, so plenty of water intake goes a long way in reducing the severity and occurrence of hay fever attacks.

Treatments: One of the best treatments for this type of congestion is the use of a nasal cleanse, such as the neti pot. When dander or pollen is the culprit, a nasal cleanse can often rinse the offending source right away, providing instant and lasting relief. This is most effective in cases when the attack can be linked to direct exposure to allergens.

Studies show that diets rich in garlic and onions contain anti-inflammatory quercetin, which can lesson or prevent the attacks. These herbs can be taken in capsule form, but are best taken directly through the diet.

Peppermint oil and other mint oils rich in menthol can help to promote the feeling of clearer breathing. While they do not actually increase the airflow, they bring about relief when diffused in the room. To use, place 1-2 drops of oil in a pot of warm water over a warm stove or dilute 1-2 drops of oil into 1 teaspoon of carrier oil and place in a shallow dish. The oil evaporates quickly and will disperse throughout the room.

Headache

What is it? A headache is another catch all term, this time referring to a painful condition in the head. This can include anything from a temporary ache from a busy day with lots of children to a serious migraine that causes sensitivity to light and sound. However, it has been estimated that 90% of headaches are tension related, which tend to begin in the back of the neck, spreading outward so, despite the numerous causes, we have a great starting point for our treatment.

Prevention: Each type of headache is the result of a different trigger, so prevention is as specific as determining which type of headache an individual is prone to experience, and eliminating that specific trigger. A little detective work is required here, but the acquired information is invaluable.

Another prevention measure is to increase the intake of magnesium. Many dietitians suggest raising the RDA of magnesium to 600 mg / day for those that are prone to headaches.

Treatments: Feverfew offers reliable relief for headaches in 2 of 3 patients that take it, according to studies. What makes it even better as a remedy is that it is also effective at offering relief for those that suffer from migraines. Pregnant women, however, should avoid the herb.

Germany's Commission E lists willow bark as an effective remedy, which makes perfect sense considering that willow bark is the source of our over the counter remedy: aspirin. They recommend 60-120mg. (The dosing is for salicin, the active compound.)

Garlic finds itself valuable again as an effective headache remedy. The platelet cells involved in blood clotting are also involved in triggering migraines. While these platelets are important to us, as they keep us from bleeding to death, we can also effectively slow down their actions. Garlic can be added liberally to the diet or taken in capsule form for these benefits.

Gingko helps to increase blood flow to the brain, which can also help to prevent headaches, especially those that occur from too much mental stimulation.

Essential oils also help to relieve headaches, and are even more effective when combined with a simple facial massage. Peppermint and lavender are my first choices. To apply, dilute 1-2 drops of the oil into 2 tablespoons of carrier oil. Olive oil and grapeseed oil are good choices, as is unscented coconut oil. (Or, try the peppermint pick me up recipe below) Then, apply to the temples of the head. Rub the thumbs across the eyebrows, lingering as you reach the center. Repeat 2-3 times or as desired. These blended oils can be prepared in advance and kept on hand (properly labeled) for situations that are likely to trigger a headache. Caution should be taken, however not to use too much essential oil. Less is always more with these potent oils, and while a small amount brings about relief, larger amounts can actually trigger headaches, which is obviously not what we are aiming for!

Peppermint Pick-Me-Up
2 T coconut oil, virgin
1 T grapeseed oil
18 drops peppermint oil
In a medium bowl, mix together your oils, making sure they are well blended. Coconut oil is a solid oil with a very low melting point, so the finished product will have a thick creamy texture that penetrates the skin quickly. Store it in a small glass vial to carry around in your first aid kit or bag.

Heartburn

What is it? Heartburn occurs when a burning pain in the chest commences after consuming a meal. This can occur to any individual infrequently, but when frequent attacks begin, a trip to the family physician is in order to look for an underlying cause.

Prevention: One of the best preventative measures we can take for our health is to sit still and relax while enjoying our daily meals. Studies show time and time again that digestion is inhibited by stress, emotional disturbances and rushing through the meal. This allows the food to sit undigested, leading to further health complications.

Treatments: Chamomile is a fantastic digestive aid, and can help to lessen the intensity of heartburn and prevent it from happening, when taken regularly after meals. It is well suited to be taken as a warm herb tea with a bit of honey or juice as a sweetener and is safe and gentle enough for all ages.

Peppermint has been used for many years as a digestive aid, taken after a meal, which has led to our modern "after dinner mint". It can be taken as a tea or enteric coated tablet for relief.

Hemorrhoids

What is it? Hemorrhoids are varicose veins in the rectum. They often result from straining too much during elimination, pregnancy, chronic constipation or diarrhea. Symptoms include pain at the affected area, bleeding during a bowel movement, tenderness and itching.

Prevention: The best prevention is to maintain a healthy diet, ensuring that stools are the correct texture to be eliminated without much difficulty. In addition to diet, a great way to ensure this happens is to always "go" when we feel the need to "go", rather than attempting to hold it in. A good general rule is to aim for one "output" with each "input" or meal.

Treatments: Treatment is aimed at reducing the symptoms and inflammation, providing relief. Instant relief can often be achieved with a soak in a warm Epsom salts bath.

Astringent herbs also help soothe the area. Witch hazel is a common herbal extract and the Thayers brand is easy to find at most drugstores. This can be kept in the bathroom and applied topically after each movement to ensure the area is thoroughly cleansed and provide quick relief, as symptoms are often intensified after a movement.

Anti-inflammatory balms and salves are also beneficial at reducing the discomfort. Calendula or chamomile balms are easy to find or make at home and can also be applied directly to the affected area, immediately after a trip to the restroom.

Hypertension

What is it? Hypertension, also referred to as high blood pressure simply means that the blood pressure reading remains consistently over 140/90, which is higher than the average of 120/80. Each time the heart beats, it pumps out blood; the higher number is when the heart pumps out the blood and the lower number is the pressure when the heart breaks between pumping.

While there are little to no symptoms, hypertension can lead to a stroke, heart failure and other serious problems, which is how it has earned the nickname as the "silent killer".

In the US, over 10 billion dollars are spent annually on anti-hypertension medications. Over half of these patients have only borderline or moderately high blood pressure readings, and studies suggest that for these individuals, nondrug therapies are the superior method of treatment. Nearly every medical authority today has a recommendation for nondrug therapies as the first line of treatment.

Prevention: Since hypertension is largely a result of lifestyle, the best prevention is a change in our modern lifestyles.

Studies show that vegetarians are less likely to have hypertension. While meat products certainly offer some nutritional benefits, our modern "meat and three" diet is packed with far more animal products that we need for a healthy diet.

Caffeine is another dietary factor. While caffeine has its benefits for some, those at risk for hypertension would do well to avoid the substance, as it can elevate the blood pressure.

Other risk factors include inactivity, stress, smoking, poor diet and nutritional deficiencies.

Treatments: First, we have to clarify that those with true hypertension might benefit from short term treatment with prescription medication to bring the numbers down while the lifestyle changes have time to be adapted and bring about their own benefits. Coming off of such a medication is something to undertake slowly and under close supervision of a licensed physician and holistic professional.

Garlic is an essential therapy for those with hypertension. It not only lowers blood pressure, but cholesterol as well, which is an added benefit, since the two are often seen together. Varro Taylor, dean and professor at Purdue University tells us that as little as a half a clove of garlic a week can reduce blood pressure. Germany's Commission E recommends 4 mg a day of fresh garlic or its equivalent. In lieu of fresh garlic, odorless capsules are available, offering similar benefits without the potential for harsh breath. Likewise, onions contain many of the same active compounds that are found in garlic, so a diet rich in these two foods offer great benefit.

Hawthorne is an herbal remedy that dilates the blood vessels, allowing more room and reducing the pressure. While it is an effective remedy, results can take up to 4-6 months to appear.

Many vegetables contain compounds that help to lower blood pressure as well. The addition of these foods to the diet would benefit anyone suffering from hypertension. These foods include (but are not limited to) celery, broccoli, tomatoes, carrots, fennel, oregano, black pepper and basil. In animal studies, the equivalent of four ribs of celery added to the diet brought about a 12-14% reduction in blood pressure. Results can be seen in as little as a week.

Insomnia

What is it? Individuals of all ages have trouble getting to sleep, staying asleep and getting enough rest while asleep. For some, especially children, this can be caused by overexcitement about the day's (or tomorrow's) activities, but the problem can appear without any obvious cause as well.

Prevention: Sticking to a routine helps the body to fall asleep at the same time each night and get plenty of rest during that timeframe. Other times, stress or a change in time zones may be the culprit and these are things that are often out of our control.

Treatments: Historically, chamomile tea was used to treat mild insomnia, preparing the body for a restful night's sleep. A cup of warm tea at bedtime is a great new habit to develop.

Valerian is a reliable sedative, but should not be taken unless the individual is fully ready to fall asleep. For children, this is a last resort, as it is a strong sedative, although still quite safe. A tincture or glycerite of the herb can be added to the chamomile tea to make it a bit more potent, or a small sip of juice for non-tea drinkers.

Melatonin is an effective remedy for insomnia due to changes in the time zones. It is not an herbal supplement, but is natural and works well. Most doses readily available are very large, and contain much more than the body naturally produces on its own (which is less than 0.3 mg a day). When we use melatonin, I chop the pills in half or even quarters for more appropriate doses. If too much melatonin is taken, it can cause restless sleep, so it is important not to take too much.

Irritability

What is it? Irritability needs no explanation, as anyone of us (that is willing to be truthful) has experienced it at one point or another. Technically speaking, irritability is an excessive response to stimuli. This can be due to many underlying problems, including headache, fatigue, stress, and many hormonal disorders. Constant irritability should alert an individual that perhaps he or she should seek professional help to learn how to better deal with the everyday ups and downs of life. However, short term irritability is generally nothing to cause a medical concern, though is certainly does pose a problem for those that we live with!

Prevention: The best way to prevent irritability is to learn how to effectively deal with stress. Every lifestyle inevitably deals with a certain amount of stress, and we have dealt with various stressors since the beginning of life outside of the Garden. It is a myth to assume that stress is a modern invention, although I would certainly suggest we have become less capable of dealing with our daily troubles.

Plenty of exercise, a healthy, whole foods diet, and a rest day each week help to prevent stress from becoming a burden in our lives.

Treatments: I would venture a guess that over half of our irritability is accompanied by a headache. Treating the headache with remedies form the headache section of this book will help alleviate some of the problem.

Excessive caffeine in the body can exhaust the adrenal glands, which can lead to anxiety and irritability. By maintaining caffeinated beverages as a balanced part of the diet in healthy individuals (or omit from the diet in some individuals), irritability can often be diminished, once the initial withdrawal symptoms have passed.

Aromatherapy plays a critical role in the treatment of irritability. Oils such as bergamot, clary sage, geranium, lavender, lemon, neroli, peppermint, sweet orange, rose, sandalwood and ylang ylang offer relaxing properties that can combat stress, treat irritability, reduce tension and balance the emotional state. They can be diffused throughout a room individually or blended to create synergesic blends. They should not, however, be applied directly to the skin.

Irritable Bowel Syndrome

What is it? Irritable bowel syndrome (IBS) has gone by many different names, including spastic colon, spastic bowel, nervous colon, nervous indigestion and functional dyspepsia. Individuals with IBS seem to have colons that are more sensitive, which creates irregular contractions instead of the normal, rhythmic ones.

Symptoms include loose stools, passage of mucus with stool, bloating, abdominal pain and altered bowel habits. Fatty foods and stress can increase these the intensity of these symptoms, especially the diarrhea, cramping and sudden urge to "go".

Prevention: When tested, over half of individuals with IBS were found to have feed sensitivities or allergies, so an elimination diet or sensitivity test can help determine these factors ahead of time.

High fiber diets have also been found to prevent and treat IBS. It is important to obtain this fiber from fruits and vegetable sources, rather than cereals and grains, since wheat and other grains are often found in combination with malabsorption and food sensitivities.

Treatments: In any intestinal problem, the first line of defense is in the form of a high quality probiotic. Proper intestinal flora is crucial in the health of the intestines and these imbalances can often be treated or prevented effectively with nothing other than a quality probiotic, which can correct these imbalances.

Peppermint oil is a reliable treatment for IBS and has been used as a digestive aid throughout history. It is still seen in some regions in the form of an "after dinner mint". Peppermint works by inhibiting smooth gastrointestinal muscle action, but when the menthol that provides this action is absorbed too early, it can lead to the relaxing of the esophageal muscle, which leads to reflux or heartburn. For this reason, enteric coated tablets are recommended, which can ensure the benefits are released at the proper point in digestion. According to trials, enteric coated peppermint tablets brought relief to over 75% of patients within two weeks.

Other common intestinal treatments include digestive enzyme supplementation and omega 3 fatty acid supplementation. Enzymes help to ensure that our food is properly digested, preventing many intestinal upsets, and omega 3 fatty acids provide anti-inflammatory benefits to the whole body.

Impetigo

What is it? Impetigo is a bacterial skin infection that usually appears as red sores around the face and mouth. The sores may appear to be full of fluid and often ooze fluid, which then forms a brownish crust over the affected area. They are usually itchy but painless and heal without scarring. Impetigo is most commonly seen in children and is highly contagious.

If the infection is accompanied by a cough or fever, or symptoms are not improving within 2-3 days, a trip to the family physician is in order.

Prevention: The infection is usually transferred through damaged skin, so close attention to cuts and scrapes will often be beneficial, especially if we know the child has been exposed, although the bacteria known to cause impetigo can also live harmlessly on the skin.

Treatments: Echinacea is beneficial for impetigo both as an internal immune booster and a topical treatment. For children, a glycerite extract is ideal regardless of the application.

Since the infection is on the skin, but beneath the crusty covering, the key to treatment is to get the antimicrobial herbs directly to the infection. To accomplish this, the affected area can be soaked with a warm, damp washcloth until the covering has been removed. Then, an ointment containing goldenseal, Oregon grape root, myrrh oil or tea tree oil is applied directly to the sores for maximum benefit. This treatment can be applied 3-4 times a day until the sores have completely healed. If making a homemade ointment, remember that alcohol extracts and pure essential oils are not to be used undiluted on a child's skin.

Jaundice

What is it? In the womb, babies receive their oxygen from red blood cells. Since they are not obtaining their oxygen from the air the same way we do, they have an abundance of red blood cells in the body to provide for their needs. After birth, however these need to be processed and eliminated. A byproduct of this change is called bilirubin, which is a yellow color. When bilirubin is not eliminated efficiently, it alters the skin color, changing it to the yellow color we associate with physiological jaundice.

Physiological jaundice will usually appear around day 2-3 of the baby's life, peaking then fading away by the end of the first week. If jaundice is accompanied by lethargy, irritability, high pitched crying, vomiting or lack of muscle tone, the advice of a physician should be sought before treating at home. A quick blood test can measure the bilirubin levels to determine whether or not advanced medical care is necessary.

There are two other types of jaundice. Breast milk jaundice appears anywhere from the end of the first week to the end of the second and usually clears up by the tenth week. In the absence of additional symptoms, this is usually fine and should not affect the breastfeeding relationship, which can and should be continued. Pathologic jaundice is usually a result of a damaged liver or infection. Jaundice that appears within the first twenty fours after birth or is not responding well with home treatment should be taken to a physician for immediate medical attention.

Prevention: Mothers that do not consume a healthy diet during pregnancy, that give birth prematurely and that take medication during labor are all more likely to give birth to an infant that becomes jaundiced.

Infants that receive plenty of sunshine after birth are less likely to become jaundiced and exposure to sunlight during the first week is generally recommended to both treat and prevent jaundice. Of course, common sense precautions should be taken. A brand new baby's skin is tender and delicate and should not receive too much sun exposure!

Breastfeeding should begin within the first hour of the baby's life when at all possible. Frequent nursing helps to ensure not only a good milk supply, but a healthy intestinal flora for baby, which can help reduce the incidence of jaundice.

Treatments: Jaundice rarely requires more than some sunlight and breastmilk, but when it does, milk thistle is my herb of choice. During my last pregnancy, I began milk thistle once I was full term and continued through the first couple of weeks. He was my only child to avoid jaundice. Milk thistle can also be given to the baby, but I usually recommend against it. It is best given to mommy, who can pass it along to baby through her milk, and I personally dislike giving anything other than breastmilk to infants younger than 6 months, per the World Health Organization's recommendation.

Jock Itch

***see Athlete's Foot**

Laryngitis

What is it? Overuse of our voice box, also known as the larynx, can lead to inflammation, which results in what we call laryngitis. Certain viral infections can also lead to this inflammation, which distorts the sound as it passes through, causing it to sound faint or even hoarse.

This is generally a short term complication, but if it persists or is accompanied by other symptoms, such as a fever, a trip to the family physician is in order to rule out other causes which are rare, but can be serious.

Prevention: The best way to avoid laryngitis is to avoid overextending the voice, giving it a rest during exciting ball games and other such activities. Plenty of fluids help as well, but clearing the throat can irritate it further.

Treatments: The first course of action is to give the voice a rest for a while. Slippery elm bark tablets can provide soothing relief through the mucilage content, but it needs to be directly applied to the throat by slowly dissolving the tablet in the mouth, allowing for maximum absorption. Marshmallow root provides similar properties and is a good substitute for slippery elm.

Horehound is also a centuries old treatment and carries the endorsement of Germany's Commission E. Little candies known as lozenges provide a fun way of treating laryngitis.

Libido, lack of

What is it? Every now and then, I answer the phone to hear a hushed voice on the other end asking me if I can help with a "small, ahem, problem". Right away I know what the call is about, and usually the caller is happy to hear that she is not the first to ask such a question! Considering the trepidation they usually have, I always wonder just how many women face the same problem yet never ask for help.

What was previously referred to as frigidity has taken on a new, kinder name "loss of libido". It often happens in females after childbearing. This can be a result of hormonal changes during breastfeeding, mild depression (or antidepressants), or simply as result of fatigue after caring for children all day.

Prevention: One of the predominant causes of loss of libido in women is pharmaceutical drug use. A common side effect is inhibited desire, yet many tend to gloss over this on the drug fact sheet, and many more never even notice that it was there. Avoiding such medications unless absolutely necessary can play a big role in preventing or treating the problem.

Treatments: Reliable aphrodisiacs have been in high demand since the beginning of time. Women from ancient cultures would seek them out for proposed benefits, often in the hopes of bearing a child. Yet, for every reliable option, there are several urban legends, and few have the time or inclination to sift through them.

Ginseng has been used as an aphrodisiac for men for many years, but many experts also report that women experience the same effects. Considering how beneficial the herb is in other areas, it is worth a try.

Anise contains phytoestrogens, plant versions of estrogens, which are thought by many experts to be responsible for libido in women. The herb can be taken as an addition to the diet for best results. For even more benefit, consider some anise flavored chocolate, see below for more on that.

It seems some men had it right all along. Not only does chocolate help beg forgiveness or win a few brownie points, it contains chemicals that relive pain and boost the mood. Endorphins and serotonin are enhanced, which can help alleviate any stressfulness that might be the culprit. It also might help explain why stressed out women tend to turn to chocolate to drown away their troubles.

Fenugreek was actually fed to women in harems to increase breast size. It also helps to alleviate hormonal problems in menopausal women, which can then in turn, prevent or alleviate the hormonal related loss of libido.

Fennel has been shown to increase libido in both male and female rats, and according to James Duke, PhD, has compounds that have been used for years to increase milk production. It is best consumed as a food, not supplement, and the oil should never be taken internally or by pregnant women.

Aromatherapy offers many herbal oils that are known aphrodisiacs. Jasmine oil is expensive and difficult to find, but highly effective oil and can be substituted with more cost friendly ylang ylang oil. When using essential oils, it is important to only purchase high quality oils, as many oils are commonly adulterated and / or diluted. Other oils include clary sage and rose. Rose is also an expensive oil that is not easy to find, but clary sage should be available at a health food store. When using essential oils, they should never be placed undiluted on the skin. Instead, dilute 2-3 drops of oil into 1 tablespoon of coconut oil for a relaxing massage or drop 1-2 drops of the blend onto a diffuser to spread throughout the room.

Lice

What is it? Lice is the plural form of louse, which is a tiny, wingless parasite which can live off of small amounts of blood drawn from the scalp. They are not dangerous, but can be quite annoying and are highly contagious.

Specifics aside, no mother enjoys the thought of tiny bugs embedded in her child's head! The bites are often itchy and scratching can lead to inflammation and even infection.

Prevention: Children can be taught how to avoid head to head contact with others. Sharing brushes, hats, scarves and other items that come in close contact with the head can contribute to the spread of lice, so keeping these items to ourselves is a great way to inhibit the spread of lice throughout a school or group.

Treatments: A study in India shows that neem oil and turmeric powder can be combined to form an effective treatment. Neem oil has a strong potent odor, but the effectiveness is worth consideration.

Tea tree oil can also get rid of the "nits" and prevent a re-occurrence, which is often common as many conventional treatments, only make them dormant for a few weeks. It is too potent to apply directly to the scalp, but 3-4 drops mixed in with the shampoo applied daily is generally enough.

Macular Degeneration

What is it? Macular degeneration is often called age relation macular degeneration or ARMD. It is the leading cause of vision loss and even blindness for adults over the age of 65 years and is literally the degeneration of the macula, which is the part of the retina responsible for sharp and clear vision.

Prevention: Research shows us that sufficient intake of Vitamins A, C and D, omega 3 fatty acids and lutein can prevent and even slow ARMD. Additionally, one study shows that individuals consuming a standard diet experienced twice the ARMD as those consuming diets rich in antioxidants for at least 5 days a week.

Smoking, hypertension (high blood pressure), inactivity and obesity are all shown to increase the incidence of ARMD, so avoidance or early treatment of these conditions prevents them from leading to additional problems.

Treatments: Bilberry, a relative of the blueberry plant is a valuable plant for eye health. It is a rich source of anthocyanocides, which are antioxidants that can also be found in blueberries, cranberries, blackberries, grapes and plums. These antioxidants strengthen the capillaries of the retina and have been found in studies to improve night vision and enlarge the visual field in participants. For best results, extracts should be standardized to contain 25% or more anthocyanidins.

Our memory herb, gingko works by improving blood flow to the brain, but it also increases blood flow to the retina. In studies, those taking gingko supplementation reported significant improvement in long distance vision and some studies even suggest gingko can reverse existing macular degeneration.

Memory Loss

What is it? One of the first signs of aging is memory loss. While young, facts and figures seem to stick so well, but as we get older, these little details seem to be more and more difficult to hold on to.

There are actually two steps to memory, we have to not only store the information in our brains somewhere, we also have to retrieve this information when we need it most. The trouble most us have is not in storage capacity, but the retrieval process. I run into this often when I hold a Q&A session after seminars. When an unrelated question comes up, I may be able to offer a handful of suggestions, but usually walk away remembering many more options that I wish I had thought of during the session. This sort of memory loss is actually said to be caused by the cumulative effect of storing additional data in the brain over many years.

Other types of memory loss are said to be a result of the decline in the amount of neurotransmitters, which are the brain's chemical messengers.

Prevention: Many factors are involved in healthy brain functioning. Most notably, a whole foods diet ensures that there is not a nutrient deficiency, which could worsen the situation and omega 3 fatty acids help to prevent loss of mental clarity.

Treatments: Gingko has been used for many years to enhance cognitive functioning. The herb improves blood flow to the brain, and has even been used to treat Alzheimer's and dementia.

Ginseng, an adaptogen, is used to normalize many functions of the body, including the response to stress and cognitive ability. Not only does it improve memory, it boosts energy levels and immune function, providing multiple benefits for aging individuals.

Menopause

What is it? The natural functions of the female body are quite fascinating when we really stop to consider things. During our "prime years", our bodies prepare for childbirth each month, constantly ready to nourish and grow a new life. When this does not happen, the body immediately starts over, preparing for the next opportunity. When a baby is conceived, the body welcomes it, cares for it and provides for its every need for nine months until it is ready to leave the womb. Then, instinctively, the body gently prepares for the exit and releases the baby into the world, once again, immediately changing gears to recovery and preparation for the next round. As if this is not amazing enough, when the body ages past the point of conceiving a child, the body naturally ceases that function in a slow and gentle process. Truly we were fearfully and wonderfully made.

Yet, this process is no longer seen as miraculous as it has been at times in history. Instead, each of these markers in the female life are treated as a problem, signs that intervention is necessary for health. We treat pregnancy as an illness, birth as a disaster waiting to happen and menopause may as well be the plague.

While it is certainly true that these changes can be uncomfortable, it is also important to remember that they are all part of a master plan. The most common symptoms include irregular cycles, more intense PMS symptoms, thinning of hair and vaginal dryness. Hormonal changes also lead to an increased risk of osteoporosis. "Hot flashes" are common, and are usually worsened or triggered by stress. These symptoms usually begin between the ages of 35 and 50, most commonly during the late forties. Sometimes the change happens quickly, yet for others, it can take several years for menstruation to completely cease.

Prevention: Every woman will eventually go through menopause, so there is no effective prevention of "the change". However, we do know that certain individuals are much less likely to experience the discomforts that are so common today.

Those that consume primarily vegetarian diets rich in beans and legumes rarely experience hot flashes or other symptoms. This is contributed to the phytoestrogens that are naturally occurring in these foods that can adhere to the estrogen receptor sites in the body. These phytoestrogens do not increase the risk of breast or reproductive system cancers and autoimmune disorders like hormone replacement therapies do.

Treatments: Considering the benefits available in phytoestrogens, food containing these substances can be liberally added to the diet for a reduction in symptoms. Soy should always be organic, as it is commonly genetically modified. Other beans and legumes also contain phytoestrogens.

Black cohosh has been shown to reduce the symptoms, specifically including hot flashes and vaginal dryness. It mimic estrogen in the body, which also contributes to its ability to reduce the depression that often accompanies menopause. It is not suitable for pregnancy or breastfeeding. Typical dose is 15-25 drops of a standard 1:5 tincture up to three times a day.

Dong quai is a Chinese herb that has been used for female complaints successfully for years and is the most common herb in Chinese medicine for this purpose.

Red raspberry leaf is the traditional midwives' remedy for any uterine function, including pregnancy childbirth and menopause. It helps to prevent the excessive bleeding that can happen during menopause and strengthens the uterus. Two to three cups of tea are generally enough for one day.

Molluscum Contagiosum

What is it? Molluscum is a viral infection that primarily affects children. It results in small pox like sores that usually appear to be filled with fluid, and closely resemble some forms of acne. These bumps or papules should not be "popped" however, as this leads to the spread of the virus to surrounding areas of skin.

The virus is extremely contagious, spreading from person to person through direct contact with contaminated objects, which can include doorknobs and toys. In adults, it can also be sexually transmitted, appearing in the genital region.

The papules typically last ten to twelve months and then clear up on their own. Some individuals, however, have experienced symptoms lasting up to four and even five years.

Prevention: Viral illnesses that spread rapidly among children are usually prevented by ensuring the child has a healthy diet, and reduce sugar intake prior to and during play groups and other times of increased exposure to common viruses. A healthy cleaning spray that removes germs but does not attempt to sterile the toy is also beneficial for moms of young children to keep on hand for these occasions.

Treatments: The functioning of the immune system has been sited as a determining factor in the healing time for children with molluscum. Generally speaking, those with decreased or sluggish immune functioning can expect to deal with the papules longer than those with healthier immune function. Therefore, adding immune boosting herbs to the routine during this viral infection can be beneficial in fighting it off from the inside out.

Topical treatment of molluscum can be difficult, since the infection lies protected within the covering of the papules and when burst, is released to spread to other parts of the body. This thick covering generally means that topical treatments can take longer to penetrate than we usually prefer, and the healing time will be directly related to the size of the papule.

Antiviral remedies that have successfully treated molluscum include tea tree oil, eucalyptus oil, and garlic oil. These can be blended to form a potent treatment suitable for tender young skin. As the skin begins to heal, the papules may begin to form a crust over the top and then fall off. Since we know that bursting the papules leads to the spread of the virus, it is important to allow this to happen naturally. Smaller papules are generally cleared up within a month, while larger ones might take up to 8 or even 10 weeks to be fully eradicated.

Antiviral Oil
In a small vial, blend 1 teaspoon garlic oil with 1/2 teaspoon tea tree oil and 1/2 teaspoon eucalyptus oil. Dilute with 1/2 teaspoon olive oil. This oil is also generally successful with warts and other viral skin conditions.

Morning Sickness

What is it? Morning sickness is the term given to the nausea experienced by expecting mothers. While the name implies something that may come and go early in the day, any experienced mother can tell you morning sickness attacks at any hour of the day, and can often be quite miserable.

Morning sickness has been linked to many different causes including low blood sugar, sluggish liver and nutritional deficiencies. Each pregnancy can affect a mother differently and even the mother that seems to always avoid it can be susceptible the next time around.

Prevention: Many a midwife has prescribed a stash of peanut butter crackers by the bed for midnight snacking to keep the blood sugar up until breakfast. This and other light protein filled snacks throughout the day are all great at preventing morning sickness that is caused by low blood sugar. The average pregnant mother needs about 80-100 grams of protein in a day, so if nothing else, this routine helps to achieve that.

Treatments: My absolute favorite remedy is the simple liver supportive herb, milk thistle. By boosting the liver to eliminate toxins and excess hormones from the body, many women experience relief. I personally used this treatment during my last pregnancy, having never experienced morning sickness before, after I experienced such nausea that I could not get out of bed until after noon on most days. Within days of beginning milk thistle three times a day, I was back to normal, yet still less than 9 weeks along. For the next 6 weeks, if I missed as little as one dose, it began to return. The best part about milk thistle is that it is perfectly safe, with no risks to the baby.

Ginger is a common anti-nausea treatment, but I do always feel the need to caution against taking too much of it. The best way to enjoy the benefits of this her is to drink real ginger ale, if the mother can stand the strong taste. Otherwise, a mild ginger tea is suitable, but not for frequent use as large amounts of the herb are said to cause miscarriage.

Chamomile helps to relieve digestion, which is sometimes the culprit, especially if the morning sickness is infrequent. Chamomile tea is the ideal form of treatment for pregnancy.

Aromatherapy oils also help relive nausea and are safe and gentle treatments for a pregnancy. Peppermint, spearmint and lemon are all beneficial. An aromatherapy diffuser is the ideal method of enjoying these oils, but in the absence of one, 3-4 drops of the oil can be added to a pot of water on a warm stove. Or, lemon slices can be placed into the glass of water that the mommy to be should be drinking plenty of, and the oils are released when she drinks. Peppermint is a strong oil, and may be too intense for early pregnancy. If this is the case, spearmint is a great way to enjoy the more gentle side of the mint family.

Nausea / Vomiting

What is it? Nausea is the feeling of discomfort and uneasiness in the stomach. More accurately, nausea is the intense gripping sensation in the stomach that is perhaps one of the worst symptoms an individual can experience. Vomiting is when that nausea wins and the contents of our stomach, along with some hydrochloric acid are viciously launched into the nearest toilet.

Nausea is a symptom, not an illness, and can be caused by many things, including an early pregnancy, food poisoning from a trip to some exotic land, or the reminder of last night's overindulgence of alcohol.

Often, simply giving in to the feeling to purge brings about sufficient relief, and, when we are not personally experiencing the pains of nausea or vomiting, we can usually see the purpose of allowing the body to eliminate whatever has triggered this reaction.

Yet, if it continues without much relief after a good vomit (is there such thing as a good vomit?), then it is time for some action. However, if it lasts longer than 24 hours, or the individual is no longer keeping fluids down and has not urinated in more than 6 hours, it is time to call the family physician to check for dehydration. This is important for all of us, but even more critical for our little ones as their bodies seem to empty much more readily than ours do.

Prevention: The best way to prevent nausea and vomiting is to avoid drinking the water in most foreign countries, to ensure that our food has been prepared in a clean manner and to avoid those that are ill with a "stomach bug".

Treatments: The first step in treating vomiting is to add fluids to the diet to prevent dehydration. I don't like the use of our conventional electrolyte drinks, as they usually contain artificial sugars and colors / flavors, which are never beneficial for an illness. Instead I like to make my own (look for a recipe under Diarrhea) or buy natural electrolyte drinks that obtain their sweetness, color and flavor from small amounts of fruit juice.

Ginger is highly effective at treating nausea and vomiting, and research shows it to be as effective as prescription medications given for nausea related to chemotherapy. If an individual is undergoing chemotherapy, it is important to first ensure that the blood clotting is not impaired. If so, ginger should be avoided.

Cinnamon contains catechins, which help to relieve nausea. It can be liberally added to food for gentle treatment. My personal favorite is some homemade applesauce with plenty of cinnamon. If taken as a supplement, cinnamon can also lower blood sugar, so diabetics or hypoglycemics should consult with a professional prior to treatment.

Peppermint contains properties that actually halt the cramping actions that lead to nausea or vomiting. It can be taken in a tea, but if there is difficulty keeping that down long enough, peppermint candies make a great substitute. The essential oil also helps to relive nausea, as discussed in the morning sickness section.

Osteoporosis

What is it? Osteoporosis literally means "porous bones". This condition, which affects women (especially after menopause) more often than men, is one that is often heavily debated. Experts agree that the bones tend to lose bone mass after around 40 years of age, but cannot agree on just how much loss is normal and at what point this loss becomes abnormal, earning the diagnosis.

Osteoporosis is actually more than a lack of calcium in the body, as commonly thought. It is the cumulative result of lack of multiple minerals and loss of framework in the bones.

Prevention: A diet rich in vital minerals is the best way to prevent a deficiency of those minerals. Abundant exercise is also shown to help prevent osteoporosis, among numerous other health concerns, and some experts go so far as suggest that activity levels are more important than diet in prevention.

There is a great deal of evidence that the phosphate in soft drinks and other foods contribute to lower bone density. Eliminating these foods and drinks from the diet certainly carries no risks with it, and considering the potential benefits, might be worth a shot.

There is also evidence pointing towards high protein diets as a risk factor for bone density loss. The body requires certain minerals to process extra protein, which can lead to fewer mineral stores in the body. The suggested daily intake for protein is consistently lowering, and many experts believe we are consuming too much. For those that are not pregnant, body builders and growing children, it might be a good idea to reconsider the ratio of fats, carbohydrates and proteins in our diet.

Treatments: Foods such as spinach, kale, broccoli, legumes, nuts and seeds are all rich in minerals and are available in the form best utilized by the body. Generally speaking, a whole foods diet, rich in fresh fruits and vegetables and occasional intake of animal products is ideal for both treating and preventing osteoporosis.

Supplementation with phytoestrogens is also beneficial for women during and after menopause, since we know there is a direct link between the two. Fermented soy is a great source of these estrogens. Additionally, cabbage and dandelion are great sources of boron, which helps to increase the estrogen levels in the blood. These can both be added liberally to any good salad, but I always feel the need to caution against picking wild dandelions. These beneficial plants are not as desirable in our lawns as they are in the medicine chest, which leads to an abundance of chemical sprays to assist in their demise. These residues are not appropriate for consumption, so growing organic dandelions or purchasing them from a reputable source is the ideal method of obtaining these small plants.

Calcium supplementation is critical to any treatment plan, but it is important to stick with a supplement that the body can actually use. Calcium citrate is ideal for maximum absorption, and Vitamin D can assist the body by increasing the absorption as well, so plenty of fresh sunshine or a multivitamin with plenty of Vitamin D will be beneficial.

Pink Eye

***see Conjunctivitis**

Poison Ivy / Oak

What is it? Poison ivy and poison oak are exactly what they sound like, plants that cause reactions in sensitive individuals. The culprit is actually urushiol, which is found in both plants, as well as poison sumac. If sensitive, a red, blistery rash appears within a few days of contact.

Prevention: It is usually difficult to be constantly vigilant about what plants we brush up against in wooded areas, but if there is a known sensitivity, keeping an eye out for these plants is always a great idea.

Treatments: Plantain offers anti-inflammatory properties that help relive the rash and irritation and reports have even made it into the *New England Journal of Medicine* about the effectiveness of the herb for poison oak and ivy. The best way to make a quick remedy from plantain is to bruise the leaves, mix them with some water and apply them directly to the affected area.

Witch hazel, the extract commonly available in pharmacies offers astringent properties that help stop the oozing and weeping of the rash. These actions feel cooling and soothing to the skin, which is a welcome change.

Cosmetic clays, such as white kaolin clay, can draw out oils from the skin, which would include the urushiol. If applied soon enough, the rash may be prevented or at least lessened, thanks to these properties.

PMS

What is it? Premenstrual Syndrome is the term given to the headache, irritability, back pain, breast tenderness, acne, food cravings and fatigue that often appear prior to the onset of one's monthly cycle. While PMS has become the brunt of many a joke, it is no laughing matter, affecting an estimated 70%-90% of menstruating women. Most experts believe that the higher estrogen levels are responsible, which would result in a direct correlation between estrogen levels and the severity of PMS.

Prevention: Many of the symptoms of PMS, especially the fatigue can be attributed to anemia. By boosting the iron stores during the month through iron rich foods, many women can effectively reduce the severity of PMS.

Many multivitamins do not contain sufficient calcium and magnesium. This can lead to decreased stores of these nutrients, which can lead to increased water retention, which in turn increases the effect of PMS symptoms.

Treatments: Evening Primrose oil is an approved treatment of PMS in many parts of Europe. Not only is it a safe and effective remedy, it is generally without side effects and offers many additional beneficial properties.

A dietary evaluation is also essential for those with moderate or severe PMS as studies show that women with these symptoms often consume a diet that is substantially worse that even the "standard American diet". It is typically high in refined carbohydrates, refined sugars and dairy, while low in most minerals. These women generally saw a dramatic reduction in symptoms after adjusting to a short term vegetarian or nearly vegan diet, reducing intake of refined products and unhealthy fats and replacing them with healthy fats and whole foods.

Milk thistle is also important in the treatment of PMS. When the liver is sluggish or stressed, it can take longer to process excess estrogen stores. By boosting the function of the liver, we can assist with this valuable function.

Prostate, enlarged

What is it? Benign prostate hyperplasia or BPH is the term given to an enlarged prostate. This common medical problem affects over 50% of men by their 60's and nearly 90% of men by their 70's or 80's. Symptoms can include a weakened urination stream, difficulty urinating, a frequent and urgent need to urinate, even at night, and urinary tract infections.

BPH is not something to self diagnose; the family physician should be consulted for a true diagnosis, as these symptoms can also be produced by more serious conditions.

When not treated, BPH can lead to rare, but serious disorders, including kidney stones and damage, more urinary tract infections and acute urinary retention. Again, these complications are rare, but not to be taken lightly.

Prevention: BPH is considered to be a result of hormonal changes due to aging, but many other contributing factors seem to play a crucial role as well. Whole foods diets with minimal pesticide intake are beneficial at preventing BPH, as are healthy cholesterol levels.

Treatments: While our first resort in the US is often pharmaceuticals, many European countries turn to botanical medications first for effective treatment.

The main ingredient in many of these remedies is saw palmetto. This extract has been clinical shown to significantly reduce the signs and symptoms of BPH. It is so effective that 90% of men in trials begin to see results in 4-6 weeks, while many pharmaceuticals can take up to a year for noticeable results. Saw palmetto helps reduce all of the symptoms listed above, but is especially beneficial at treating the nighttime urination, which leads to a better night's sleep.

Pumpkin seeds are also known to reduce the need to urinate frequently and suddenly. General dose is one tablespoon daily, but they can be taken in greater amounts as a tasty addition to the diet, or blended to make a creamy nut butter alternative.

Restless Legs Syndrome

What is it? Imagine you are relaxing on the couch after a long day. As you lay there, perfectly still, you begin to feel an overwhelming urge to move your legs. You resist, remaining still, but the urge is so strong that you begin to feel tugging, burning and itching sensations. The antsy feeling is overwhelming, and you *must* move your legs.

As bizarre as this sounds, this is exactly what it feels like to have restless legs syndrome, a neurological condition that causes an uncomfortable feeling in the legs while resting that is alleviated once the legs are exercised. It can also happen in the trunk of the body or the arms, but any location is likely to inhibit sleep, as the body cannot rest or relax while having these sensations.

Prevention: Research shows that the symptoms can be relieved by stimulating or exciting conversation, so engaging in some mental exercise prior to bedtime or any other resting time can be used to prevent the discomfort. We also know that caffeine can aggravate the symptoms, so it should be avoided by those with restless legs syndrome.

Certain nutritional deficiencies, particularly iron and folic acid, are also common among those with RLS. Ensuring that a healthy, whole foods diet, rich in B complex vitamins, vitamin C and iron can prevent or even treat RLS.

Treatments: Valerian, an herbal sedative, is effective at treating restless legs syndrome. It should not be taken unless the individual is fully ready for a good night's sleep, but when it is taken, it can help the affected individual actually fall asleep, instead of allowing the sensations to keep them up all night, which is the most common problem with RLS.

Likewise, kava kava can be taken prior to bedtime to relax the muscles and help soothe the central nervous system. It should not be taken prior to driving anywhere and should not be taken with alcohol as it can cause a feeling of inebriation and intensify the effects of any alcohol.

Ringworm

***see Athlete's Foot**

RSV

What is it? Respiratory syncytial virus causes infection of the lungs and respiratory tract (also called bronchiolitis, the name for the childhood version of bronchitis). It is extremely common, affecting most children by the age of 2 or 3. When it occurs in older children, it is usually very similar to the common cold, but when it occurs in young infants, it can be serious. The virus actually causes damage to the cells lining the air passages, leaving the lungs weakened for weeks.

Symptoms also resemble cold or flu symptoms and include runny nose, dry cough, mild fever, sore throat and discomfort. Infants however, may experience difficulty breathing and may act lethargic. In these cases, a trip to the family physician is in order.

Prevention: As any other common virus, prevention measures focus on consuming a whole foods diet, avoiding sugar intake, which can lower the immune system by up to 40% for up to 4 hours, and boosting the immune system through immune supporting herbs when in situations that lead to increased exposure, such as air travel, large parties or schoolrooms.

RSV is more common in the winter and spring, and in prematurely born infants or infants that are fed formula. Additional precautionary measures should be considered for these situations.

Treatments: As this is a viral infection, antibiotics are not only ineffective, studies actually show they can prolong the duration of the infection. Most RSV can be treated at home with supportive therapy, but it is also one of the leading causes of hospitalization among infants younger than one year.

Nighttime steam treatments form the shower are often beneficial, especially as the cough is often much worse at night. For babies older than 4-6 months, a single drop of eucalyptus essential oil diluted with a teaspoon of olive oil can be placed on the floor of the shower to waft through the room. Care should be taken not to apply this steam directly onto the baby's face.

Chamomile tea offers anti-inflammatory properties and can be beneficial for children that are old enough to drink other fluids, although breastfeeding babies should be getting plenty of breastmilk for the powerful immune boosting benefits.

Other immune boosting herbs should be continued for additional assistance as the body fights the virus, but be sure to take the age of the child into consideration before administering remedies. For babies too young for herbal supplements, mommy can take the herb in a weight appropriate dose (working on the smaller end of the dosing range) and baby will receive these benefits with the next nursing session.

Sciatica

What is it? Sciatica is the term to describe the pain that flows along the sciatic nerve from the lower back through the buttock and down the leg. This pain can range from a mild ache to a harsh, tingling, unbearable pain, and usually chooses to remain on one side of the body.

While there are many things that can cause sciatica, it is important to remember that sciatica is the symptom, not the disorder, so treatment generally involves more than simply taking a pain reliever to mask the symptom. Sciatica can be caused by trauma, a herniated disk, tumors, and I have even been told one client had sciatica simply from storing his rather large wallet in the same back pocket for many years. If the underlying cause is severe, it will require medical treatment, otherwise, most cases of sciatica clear up on their own within 8 weeks, although rare cases can persist many years.

Prevention: While the causes may vary, individuals that lead sedentary lifestyles are more likely to experience sciatica, so plenty of activity and exercise are great prevention measures.

Treatments: Chiropractic care is often all that is necessary to eliminate the painful symptoms associated with sciatica. My first line of treatment would involve enlisting the help of a reputable chiropractor.

White willow bark contains salicin, and is actually the first source of aspirin. It helps treat any pain related problem in the body, and is especially useful for back pain. Up to six 400 mg capsules can be taken in a day, but long term use, especially of higher doses, can lead to stomach irritation.

Dong quai is known as a female herb, but the anti-inflammatory, antispasmodic and mild analgesic properties make it well suited for sciatica. While it is not appropriate for pregnancy, other individuals can take it brewed into a tea or in an extract or capsule equal to 2-4g of the dried root per day.

Shingles

What is it? Shingles is a viral infection that causes a painful rash, appearing as a patch of blisters. It usually occurs on the trunk of the body, but can also involve the neck and scalp, although it typically only affects one side of the body. It is caused by the same virus that causes the chicken pox and typically affects older adults or those with weakened immune systems.

While pain is usually the first and most obvious symptom, shingles can also involve a fever, chills, headache and upset stomach. The blisters usually last 7-14 days, then form crusty scabs and fall off.

Prevention: Like most health concerns, a whole foods diet and immune support play key roles in prevention. Stress is also a factor in the outbreak of the virus, so prevention measures should be boosted during stressful situations to prevent susceptibility due to lowered immunity.

Treatments: Lemon balm is an effective treatment for cold sores, which is relevant here because cold sores are a result of a virus that comes form the same family and acts much like the virus that causes shingles. To take advantage of these benefits, a lemon balm (or *Melissa*) cream is well suited for topical application. In a health food store, it is probably located with other cold sore remedies. Lemon balm tea is a great solution to use for a topical compress to be applied directly to the affected area. Lemon balm is a part of the mint family, so other mint herbs would be great additions to a blend.

Garlic helps to boost the immune function and is effective at fighting off both viral and bacterial infections. While it can be taken as an odorless supplement, I would just add it liberally to the diet if I had shingles.

Capsicum is well-suited for topical application on painful skin irritations. From the red or cayenne pepper plant, capsicum is often used for arthritis and other inflammatory problems. While capsicum is readily available in a commercial preparation in most health food stores, it can easily be prepared by adding a powdered herb to some olive oil. For ready made creams, follow the manufacturer's directions, but for the homemade variety, rub a small dab gently into the affected area. Wash hands immediately and be sure not to get the oil into the eyes or facial area as the pepper can burn.

Licorice is well-known as a potent antiviral herb. Applied topically, it not only helps to fight the infection, it also helps to reduce inflammation, leading to a reduction in pain as well. I rarely suggest licorice in a standard extract, but for topical use, it is perfectly acceptable. It can be applied directly to the affected area in either a store bought extract or homemade licorice tea on a compress.

Mullein not only helps to inhibit the virus, it also reduces pain and inflammation. The best way to soothe irritated skin is to apply mullein in a compress made from a strong tea brewed with 1-2 teaspoons of the dried herb per 8 ounces hot water.

Aromatherapy also offers some great herbal essential oils that play a valuable role in treating viral infections. Bergamot, chamomile, lavender and lemon are all good choices. To use, blend 3-4 drops of the oil into a tablespoon of olive oil. Massage directly into the affected area(s). Repeat 2-3 times a day. Essential oils should never be taken internally.

Sick Building Syndrome

What is it? While it may sound like it came straight out of a late night comedy skit, sick building syndrome is actually quite real and affecting more and more individuals every year.

Sick building syndrome refers to the compounded affects that are caused by poor indoor air quality. This can include headache, congestion, nervous system disorders, allergies, asthma, fatigue and irritation. This of course sounds like fairly vague symptoms, but the World Health Organization has estimated that 30% of individuals worldwide are currently experiencing sick building syndrome. This could be a major contributor of all of our "unexplained" health problems.

The air inside our homes and other buildings has been listed as one of the top 5 environmental risks to our health. Many common building materials such as carpeting, pressed wood products, paints, glues and resins, draperies, and wall coverings emit toxins into the air that we breathe in day and night. As it turns out, that new home smell is not so great, after all!

Prevention: The best way to prevent sick building syndrome is to purchase, build and redecorate as naturally as possible. By using low or no VOC paints, solid wood flooring and cabinetry, installing (and actually opening and using) many windows for fresh air, and limiting our synthetic home décor products, we can safely eliminate many of the sources of sick building syndrome. Most of the time, these more natural substances are easier to maintain and add to the decorative appeal of the home, so there are added benefits to maintaining a healthy home. You can even make them yourself using some of the formulas in the Natural Family Toolkit towards the end of this book. Most of the ingredients are easy to find at the local grocer or health food store.

Treatments: The best way to treat sick building syndrome is to remove the source of the problem. Some homes tend to be more toxic than others, and this may require a major renovation of the home, which is not always possible. Others, however, may be simple solutions that are surprisingly cost effective. For example, many times a more commonly used room can be redecorated with solid wood or bamboo flooring for a major reduction in toxic outgassing. Or we can choose no VOC paints from the home improvement store for the same price as the standard kind, and this is an even better investment when we are painting a child's room or a new nursery.

When that home has been improved as much as it can be given the budgetary and time constraints of such a project, other smaller actions can still help to improve the air quality inside the house. Windows should be opened regularly to allow air flow, flushing out the old air and allowing in new air. If this is not always possible, look for ideal days, with high wind and open two windows on opposite ends of the home so that a few good gusts can bring some cleaner air inside the home.

Additionally, the products we use to clean our homes are actually making them more dirty, replacing plain dirt with toxic sludge. When we spray harsh cleaners in the home, we release harmful fumes into the air that we breathe in. We also leave chemicals on our dishes, our clothes and the surfaces of our homes. This is then ingested as our food sits on our plates prior to consumption, our clothing rubs against our bodies and our furnishings are used on a daily basis. Instead, this can be adjusted with a simple change to natural, safer cleaners. Personally, I have found that an all natural cleaner with eucalyptus oil and lemon grass is much more pleasant to clean the home with, leaves a nice aroma throughout the home and does not place my children at high risk for allergies and asthma the way conventional cleaners will.

We also place live plants strategically throughout our home to clean the air. Studies show that plants actually remove carcinogens and other toxins from the air, replacing it with clean and pure air. Formaldehyde and toluene are two common problems that are quickly removed by live plants. When tested, palms and ferns consistently ranked high on the list in terms of amount of toxin removal from the air.

Sinus Infection

What is it? Also called sinusitis, a sinus infection is a common complication of the even more common cold. This occurs when the air passages behind the bones in our cheeks, eyebrows and jaw become inflamed and infected. These passages serve as filters and actually help to protect the lungs from damage.

When a cold is on the way out, then the body suddenly takes a turn for the worse, a sinus infection is often to blame. Symptoms include facial pain, especially along the areas of the nose and forehead, stuffy nose, fever and headache that worsens when bending down.

Prevention: A sinus infection or inflammation can be triggered by use of nasal sprays (especially frequent use), smoking, swimming, and even a change in air pressure or temperature. When these factors are present, additional immune boosting measures are appropriate.

During a cold, the nasal passages can be rinsed with a nasal irrigation pot, more frequently known by the name brand neti pot. These allow a saline solution to flow through the nostrils, removing stagnant mucus, providing clearer breathing and eliminating the chance for stagnant mucus to become infected. When herbs such as Oregon grape root are added, the cleanse can actually apply antiseptic properties directly to the area, preventing or even treating infection.

Use of a neti pot generally requires a learning curve, and if used incorrectly, the saline wash can actually further aggravate sinus inflammation, so it is generally recommended than an individual practice the rinse when illness is not present so that the habit is well developed before mucus sets in. If the mucus is already thick, the rinse might not always move everything through, but the solution works to break down the mucus, diluting it so that it can be eliminated.

I also recommend the massage that is described in the ear infection section. This brings about relief from the symptoms of a stuffy nose, and can help the mucus to work its way through. It may not feel soothing for an intense infection, however, so if it does not bring about relief, discontinue its use.

Treatments: For infections, garlic is a reliable, fast working and effective herb to put to work in the body. It can be added to the diet with little trouble, and odorless capsules are readily available.

Another dietary treatment includes the consumption of spicy or "hot" foods. Cayenne pepper, horseradish and wasabi all flush the sinuses and increase breathing.

Echinacea and Oregon grape root or goldenseal make a powerful blend for fighting off infections, especially if they have a bacterial cause. In appropriate doses, it can be used for children as well, but pregnant women should avoid the use of goldenseal or Oregon grape root.

Eucalyptus and mint oils help to allow clear breathing during sinus problems. I do not recommend applying these directly to the skin, but a single drop can be added to a tablespoon of a lotion or petroleum free jelly for massage onto the chest to promote clear breathing. While this cannot be used with children, I have often placed it onto my own chest so that the child can easily breathe in the oils as I hold them.

Gingko increases the blood flow to the head, which brings the important white blood cells (also called fighter cells) to the affected area. Generally speaking, blood flow is increased naturally to infected or wounded areas in the body, but a little help brings about healing faster.

Skin Problems

What is it? We obviously use the term "skin problem" in a broad general sense here, as there are many specific skin conditions that one could experience. Most common are dry skin, eczema and allergic rashes. Eczema was tackled under its own heading, so we will not revisit that. Dry skin can be caused by a number of triggers. Anything from travel (especially air travel) to inadequate hydration to living in a dry climate or even a seasonal change of weather can lead to both short term and long term dry skin.

Body care products, laundry soap and even food products can cause reactions on the skin, and unless removed from the picture, will continue to cause problems.

Prevention: The best way to maintain beautiful skin is to drink plenty of liquids. Ideally, an individual should consume half their body weight in ounces. So, a 120 pound female would aim for 60 ounces of water daily. Certain lifestyle factors can lead to an increased need for water, however. This includes air travel, consumption of alcohol and any intense physical exercise. I generally recommend an extra 6-8 ounce glass of water for each hour in the air, each alcoholic beverage consumed and each hour of physical exercise.

Treatments: Many times, skin troubles are directly related to an irritating laundry soap or body care product. All of these things are known to contain harsh synthetic substances that can easily irritate sensitive skin. Replacing them with natural products is actually not only beneficial for the skin but quite pampering. The natural laundry soaps we use regularly in our home always make our laundry smell fresh and clean, not harsh like cheap perfume, and our natural skin care products leave our skin soft and supple with intensely rich natural scents and luxurious ingredients. In the Natural Family Toolkit towards the end of the book, there are several formulas for making natural body care products at home using ingredients from the local health food store.

Sometimes, skin inflammation is caused by an imbalance of omega 3 fatty acids to omega 6 fatty acids. Our modern diets offer plenty of omega 6 acids, but rarely enough omega 3s. To alter this, we can supplement with evening primrose oil (EPO) or fish oil. The oils are readily available in capsule form and can be taken according to the package directions. Evening primrose oil and flax oil are also great soothing oils that can bring about beneficial results through topical application as well.

Chamomile also offers plenty of anti-inflammatory properties that can help many skin problems. The best way to use chamomile is to brew a strong tea and apply the infusion as a compress onto the skin, once it has cooled. Chamomile is approved by Germany's Commission E for topical use on skin inflammation.

Calendula is another yellow flowering plant that offers benefits to the skin when applied topically. Calendula can be applied in a compress, but is often available in a cream or oil for regular use. Weleda offers an entire line of baby care with calendula that helps protect and treat their delicate skin.

Witch hazel is readily available at any local drugstore or grocer and provide astringent actions that help to reduce inflammation and enhance blood supply to affected areas. It is also approved by Germany's Commission E for inflamed skin, and considering how easy it is to locate, I would not hesitate to use it on irritated skin, especially when traveling. It is used externally by dabbing directly onto the affected area with a cotton ball. For additional benefits, the skin can then be moisturized with a calendula cream or chamomile ointment.

Smoking

What is it? Smoking is not an illness, but a habit that is often a result of an addiction to nicotine, a substance in tobacco leaves. It can lead to multiple health concerns, such as an increased risk for lung cancer and many respiratory problems.

Smoking is said to be responsible for one third of all cancer related deaths and one fourth of all fatal heart attacks in the United States. Considering that smoking does not offer any benefits to the body to make up for these risks, there really is no good reason not to kick this unhealthy habit.

Prevention: The best way to prevent a smoking habit is to avoid smoking in the first place. There really is no other prevention for an addiction to nicotine.

Treatments: Nicotine binds to certain receptor sites in the brain that affect mood, so individuals that are attempting to quit smoking, especially if going "cold turkey" have a good excuse for acting moody and slightly depressed. Yet, the habit can and should be beaten. To quit smoking requires plenty of willpower and most aids are just that, aids. They are not designed to actually remove the desire or break the habit, rather, they help provide alternatives for when that urge strikes and help to heal the damaged bodily tissues, preventing smoking-related diseases.

Many people smoke because of stress, and stress is one of the top reasons individuals turn back to smoking after making progress at quitting. So, to prevent this downfall, herbal adaptogens can help an individual cope with stressful situations in life, reducing the urge to turn back to the habit. Astragalus and holy basil are two adaptogens that are highly effective, gentle and also boost the immune system.

Valerian also helps the individual to fall asleep, especially when nighttime smoking has been the bedtime routine. It is a reliable sedative that should only be used when ready for bed, not before driving or when there is not sufficient time to devote to sleep.

Kava kava can help reduce the anxiety that is experienced during the withdrawal phase. It does not generally cause drowsiness, but when taken in excess, it can cause inebriation. Until the ideal dose is found, it should only be taken at home, when there is no need to operate a vehicle. It should not be taken by those on antidepressants, pregnant women or in combination with alcohol.

A smoking habit often depletes the body of the B complex vitamins, so supplementation with these nutrients is a good idea, especially considering what a vital role these nutrients play in the cognitive functioning.

Sore Muscles

What is it? Many of us are reluctant to admit that we are not the athletes we like to pretend we are. While our ideal life includes daily sports activities, our real lives do not always allow such luxuries. Unfortunately, this means that when we are able to get outside and play, we often push ourselves too far and end up with what has often been called the "athlete's hangover". Sore muscles, swelling, and an overall achy feeling can all be attributed to a lack of preparation for athletic events.

Prevention: Most of our problems can be linked to dehydration, so it is absolutely crucial that we drink plenty of water and electrolyte drinks before playing too hard. Vitamins, especially E and C, are also necessary for eliminating toxins that may build up and cause problems.

When a problem does occur, however, it is important to seek medical treatment for any actual injuries, and to stay calm and rest until fully healed. Contrary to popular thought, pushing through an injury does not make one tough. It can prolong the injury and increase the damage.

Treatments: Arnica is my herb of choice for any sports related soreness or swelling. It makes a great compress, but is also easy to find in a cream or ointment. It soothes inflammation and helps to heal bruises and sprains. Arnica should not be applied to open wounds or taken internally.

Peppermint provides that familiar cooling sensation on the skin (thanks to the menthol content) that brings about relief from the pain of sore muscles. Ointments containing peppermint can be found at a health food store, or an oil can be made by combining 10-15 drops of peppermint oil with an ounce of olive oil. Peppermint can irritate extremely sensitive skin, and this is magnified by heat, so before combing peppermint with heat, be sure your skin can tolerate it.

Comfrey is excellent at relieving pain, swelling, and inflammation. It is best applied topically in an ointment or salve, which can be purchased at a health food store.

Sore Throat

What is it? A sore throat really needs no explanation. Anyone that has ever had a cough, strep throat or been exposed to harsh chemicals can attest to the pain and irritation that are involved in the soreness of a sore throat.

The first sign of a cold is often a sore throat, and when I wake up with one, I always immediately begin cold treatments to prevent the cold from setting in. Usually this works and by the afternoon I am symptom-free again. When the throat is sore and there is also a fever, a trip to the family physician is in order to rule out strep throat, which should not be treated at home.

Prevention: The best way to prevent a sore throat caused by chemical exposure is to avoid breathing in stagnant air in places full of toxins such as mechanic shops or many production facilities. When these locations are a requirement of one's job or duties, well ventilated air should be provided to reduce the damage to the body.

Treatments: Many commercial throat lozenges do not actually reduce the inflammation at all, instead they release anesthetic properties to numb the nerve cells in the throat temporarily. While this certainly can reduce the discomfort, it leaves that actual problem untreated. Herbal lozenges, however actually treat and soothe the inflammation, providing short term and long term relief.

Slippery elm bark lozenges are probably the best herbal remedy for a sore throat. Thayers brand carries a wide line of flavored lozenges that are usually easy to find and taste so good that I have to hide them from my kids. These should not be chewed and swallowed quickly, as the actions need to be fully exposed to the throat to be effective. Instead, they should be allowed to dissolve slowly in the mouth.

Marshmallow contains many of the same properties that slippery elm bark does, but is well suited to a tea infusion. Generally, 2-3 teaspoons of crushed herb per cup of boiling water can be taken 2-3 times a day for relief.

Garlic may not be specifically for the throat, but is a general antiviral immune stimulant that helps the body fight off the underlying infection that is causing the problem. Not only can garlic be taken in capsules for benefits, it can be liberally added to the diet, making it an easy to find herb when traveling or out of the house, which seems to always be when these things are needed!

Licorice not only fights off viral infections, it also reduces inflammation, soothes the throat, and boosts the immune system. For ulcers, we recommend the DGL licorice (deglycyrrhizinated licorice), but for treatment of viral illness, this type is not effective and the whole herb should be used. However, this can cause problems for some people, so avoid the whole herb if you are pregnant, breastfeeding, have hypertension, diabetes, thyroid problems, heart problems, liver problems or kidney problems. Otherwise, it can be taken safely for up to 4-6 weeks.

Styes

What is it? Styes (also spelled sties) are irritating and painful infections in the glands of the eyelid. They generally last a couple of days, then go away on their own. However, once a child experiences this bacterial infection, they are more likely to experience a reoccurrence.

Prevention: Prevention of styes centers around limiting what we allow to come into contact with our eyes. Sharing cosmetics and rubbing the eyes are two common examples.

Individuals that are prone to reoccurring infections often have a vitamin A deficiency. Supplementation with this nutrient should be a part of the daily multivitamin, but the best way to get this vitamin into the body is to consume foods rich in carotene such as carrots and leafy greens.

Treatments: A warm compress with herbal tea brings about quick relief. Chamomile and eyebright are two good herbs for this. Simply infuse some dried herbs into warm water and place a cloth saturated with the tea on the closed eye. For maximum benefit, this compress can remain in place up to 20 minutes, three times a day.

Considering that many physicians prescribe antibiotics orally for styes, plenty of herbalists recommend taking echinacea as an alternative to the harsher antibiotics. I personally have always found quick relief from the warm compress with eyebright on it, but if anyone in my family experienced one that did not go away quickly, we would begin oral echinacea as both a treatment measure and preventative measure for reoccurrence. Echinacea should not be taken internally for extended periods of time, so 3-4 weeks should be sufficient.

Sunburn

What is it? Sunburn is the reddening and inflammation of the skin's outer layers as a result of overexposure to the sun's powerful rays. Compared to other burns, sunburn is generally mild, but the experience leads to an increased risk for skin cancer, and does damage to the skin, causing premature aging.

Prevention: The best prevention for sunburn is to wear sunscreen when appropriate and ensure there are plenty of layers between us and the sun during the middle of the day. We tend to have polar extremes when it comes to sunscreen. Many individuals avoid it altogether in search of the perfectly tanned skin, leading to the above mentioned damage. Others, however, tend to slather on the sunscreen and stay hidden indoors during the hottest parts of the day, which is not recommended either, as the sun provides plenty of benefits to the body as well. One prime example is with our sunshine vitamin, vitamin D. Studies show that most babies and children are now deficient in this nutrient, which increases the risk of cancer and minor problems such as the common cold. Yet, this can be prevented with only 10-15 minutes of unhindered sun exposure a day. Like many things, we are in need of some healthy balance and common sense when it comes to sun exposure.

Treatments: I will never forget the time we went to a water park and my fair skinned husband ended the day with a flaming red back and neck. Stuck in a part of the country I was entirely unfamiliar with, I had no idea how we were going to treat this, as I had not brought any burn remedies. Our solution was to head to the closest grocery or vitamin store we could find and walk the spice aisle looking for anything that might work. Sure enough, tucked away in a vitamin shop, I found a box of organic chamomile tea and some vitamin E capsules. We brewed the tea in the hotel with some hot water and applied cool compresses to his shoulders all night. The next day when we returned to the water park, his skin was back to normal. Of course, while I am grateful to have found the tea packets, we now carry an herbal first aid kit with us whenever we travel to avoid this treasure hunt next time!

Chamomile offers anti-inflammatory properties, but it also stimulates healing by closing the wounds and stimulating the growth of new cells. When combined with plenty of water, as in the tea compress, it helps to prevent dehydration and limits the damage to the skin. Calendula offers the same benefits.

Vitamin C in the diet helps to stimulate the repair of sun damaged skin. It is easy to find in some fresh fruit or orange juice, or can be taken in buffered vitamin C supplements. Likewise, essential fatty acids are crucial for tissue repair. Supplementation with fish oil or flax oil after a sunburn can speed the repair process.

Plantain is soothing to the skin, and also stimulates the growth of new skin cells. It is a great addition to a balm or salve for inflamed skin or any kind.

Witch hazel extract contains tannins, which bring about cooling relief by removing heat form the burn. It also simulates the growth of new skin cells, speeding recovery, repairing skin damage and reversing the chance of sunburn induced cancer.

Vitamin E applied topically soothes and brings relief to irritated skin, especially burned skin. Capsules can be popped open to gently massage onto the area.

Teething

What is it? Teething is the term given to the time in an infant's life when the teeth begin to break through the gums into the mouth. It causes discomfort, swelling and even pain for the baby, which can lead to irritability and sleepless nights.

In addition to the pain, teething can also cause swollen gums, drooling, mild fever, irritability, more frequent nursing (sometimes with biting!), and the overwhelming urge to chew on anything baby can get his or her hands on! Most experts agree that runny nose and fever over 101 is not associated with teething, but the stress of the situation can certainly make baby more prone to illness.

Prevention: The emergence of teeth is a milestone many parents eagerly anticipate. There are no prevention measures for this development.

Treatments: Herbs for Kids makes a topical treatment called Gum-omile, which contains clove oil and chamomile extract. This is one of my absolute favorite remedies in the home during these milestones. I have occasionally found the oil to be too strong for my younger babies, but when that happens, I simply dilute it with equal parts of olive oil.

Bach Rescue Remedy, probably the most popular of Bach's flower remedies, is effective at reducing the stress and anxiety that can be a result of teething, and also helps combat the stress and anxiety in a tired mama! For babies, 2-4 drops of the extract are generally sufficient. Mommies can follow the dosing guidelines on the package.

Chickweed also soothes inflammation, which in turn helps the process move along much smoother. A single drop or two of a glycerine extract can be massaged into the affected gums for topical treatment. Since most babies are quite young while teething, they should be observed for potential allergies anytime a new substance is introduced.

Toothache

What is it? A toothache is generally a sign of an underlying problem. Most commonly, a toothache signals that the nerves of the tooth are either dead or dying. Studies show that most individuals are hesitant to visit the dentist for a toothache, but if the problem persists, such a trip is in order, as it can potentially grow into a larger problem quickly.

Prevention: Good oral hygiene is the best prevention for such oral problems, but a healthy, whole foods diet is also a must for strong teeth that don't chip easily and gums that can resist infection.

Treatments: Clove oil is a fantastic remedy for a toothache. The oil offers antiseptic properties, which can be beneficial in the case of an infection. It also offers anesthetic properties that bring about temporary relief from the pain. It is not to be ingested, but a swab can be used to apply the diluted oil to the affected area. It should be diluted by mixing 5-6 drops of clove oil with 1 tablespoon olive oil. Mix well and store the rest for future use in a clearly labeled container.

For adults, James Duke, PhD, recommends ginger, which can make an effective remedy, but may be too intense for sensitive individuals. Since it is topically applied to the tooth, it is fairly easy to rinse off if it is too strong. Ginger relieves the pain by irritating the skin, which then reduces the underlying irritation. We call this a counter irritant. Powdered ginger can be mixed with oil in equal ratios until a paste is formed. With a swab, apply it topically to the tooth. If it burns, quickly remove by brushing the teeth and rinsing well.

Ulcers (peptic ulcers)

What is it? A peptic ulcer is a sore that is caused by the literal burning of delicate tissue by the strong digestive (acidic) juices of the stomach. This can happen in many places along the digestive tract, but occurs most often in the duodenum.

Like reflux, previous theories have included the notion that some bodies contain excessive stomach acid, but research has shown that this is not the case. Aside from individuals with tumors, the amount of stomach acid is unrelated to the occurrence of ulcers.

Another theory is that the ulcers have a bacterial cause. A bacterium, *H. plylori,* has been thought to weaken the lining of the stomach, allowing the acid to penetrate and cause harm. Yet, that has also been disputed by additional research, since many individuals have *H. plylori,* yet do not develop ulcers, and only about 50% of those with ulcers have *H. plylori.* However, it is still considered to be a contributing factor in some cases, primarily because the recurrence rate is lowered when it is eliminated.

Prevention: Prevention focuses on removing from our diet and lifestyle those things that are known to contribute to ulcers or aggravate them. This includes NSAIDs (non steroidal anti-inflammatory drugs), excessive alcohol consumption, low fiber diets, food allergies and nutritional deficiencies. It is important to realize that even moderate use of NSAIDs, such as ibuprofen or aspirin can contribute to an ulcer.

Additionally, it is interesting to learn that one physician successfully treated ulcers with nothing but water, as dehydration can lead to an increase in the occurrence, since sufficient water intake is critical for proper mucosal lining. Ensuring sufficient water intake certainly has other health benefits as well, so it definitely worth considering.

Treatments: Most intestinal problems benefit from the addition of probiotics to the routine. These beneficial strands of bacteria help maintain a healthy intestinal flora.

Digestive enzymes help to prevent undigested food from remaining in the intestines, causing further irritation and inflammation.

Cranberry extract and juice inhibit *H. plylori.* The unsweetened juice is a great daily habit, but extracts are also beneficial for those that do not enjoy the flavor.

Licorice contains ulcer inhibiting compounds that some trials have shown to be more effective than standard medical treatments, with fewer side effects. Licorice also contains a compound that can be harmful to certain individuals in long term intake of large amounts, but deglycyrrhizinated licorice, which has that compound removed has been shown to be just as effective without the side effects.

Ginger is a common digestive aid with many anti-ulcer properties. Candied ginger is a great way to enjoy these benefits.

Urinary Tract Infection

What is it? A urinary tract infection is an infection that affects any part of the urinary tract. Urine should not contain bacteria, but nearly 85% of urinary tract infections are caused by *E. coli,* which is commonly found in the intestines.

Such infections are much more common among women, partially due to the closer proximity of the urethra and anus. Symptoms include an urgent desire to empty the bladder, frequent and painful urination, spasms and the urge to urinate, although little to no urine actually comes out.

Prevention: Hygiene plays a key role in preventing urinary tract infections. Bubble baths and other bath additives as well as many feminine products can also trigger infections.

Treatments: Unsweetened cranberry juice can produce hippuric acid in the urine, which can inhibit bacterial growth and prevents the adherence of bacteria to the lining of the bladder.

A different approach involves alkalizing the urine with minerals bound to citrate (calcium citrate, for example). This works best when combined with antibacterial herbs, which require an alkaline environment for optimal performance.

An echinacea and goldenseal combination is an effective antibiotic for treating urinary tract infections. The barberine in goldenseal prevents the bacteria from adhering to the lining of the urinary tract, and provides antibacterial actions without disturbing intestinal flora. Many herb companies are now choosing to use Oregon grape root instead of goldenseal because of the possibility of endangering the botanical species. This is a reliable substitute, since they both rely on the same herbal compounds. Neither goldenseal nor Oregon grape root are suitable for pregnancy or extended treatments, however.

Uva ursi, also called bearberry, is perhaps the most useful herb in treating urinary tract infections. It carries with it not only a long historic use, but quite a bit of research demonstrating its abilities to combat *E. coli*. Another factor to consider is that this herb also dramatically reduces the re-occurrence rate of the infection, which is often fairly high. One trial reflected a 0% re-occurrence rate for those that treated the initial infection with uva ursi. The herb, however should only be taken by adults and in minimal doses, as side effects begin to occur in as little as 15 grams of dried leaf.

During an infection, foods that have adverse effects on the bladder should be avoided. This includes alcohol, sugars, processed foods and caffeine, which can cause painful spasms.

Regardless of treatment methods, an 8 ounce glass of water should be taken every hour to help clear the urinary tract and dilute the urine.

Varicose Veins

What is it? Varicose veins occur when the veins that allow the blood to flow back do not function properly, primarily because they have become weakened. They instead allow the blood to pool, and the surrounding capillaries become swollen. When this occurs near the surface of the skin, it causes visible lumps in the veins, which also show up as bluish streaks or spidery veins. This is extremely common during pregnancy as a result of the excess weight and blood flow that is occurring. As expected, these are most likely to appear on the legs, especially the upper thighs.

Prevention: Poor circulation is a contributing factor for the development of varicose veins, so individuals with lifestyles that involve plenty of sitting or standing in one place are much more likely to develop varicose veins, especially if this lifestyle is not changed after a significant weight gain or pregnancy.

Some experts also believe that birth control pills and hormone replacement therapy can contribute to the formation of varicose veins. These medications can usually be replaced with more natural, safer therapies with equal effectiveness.

Treatments: Horse chestnut helps to strengthen the veins, by sealing off tiny openings in the walls, reducing the leakage of fluid. It also helps to reduce itching and swelling. While it is highly effective, and even bears the approval of Germany's Commission E, it should only be taken if a standardized extract with clear dosing guidelines can be found, which is not as easy to do in the United States as it is elsewhere. Otherwise, skip the internal use of this herb and focus on a prepared cream for topical application. Either way, don't make your own. The herb can be quite toxic and should be prepared correctly.

Butcher's broom contains powerful anti-inflammatory compounds to reduce inflammation. It also helps to constrict and strengthen the veins, preventing the pooling that occurs within weak veins.

Witch hazel extract is an astringent, which means that it can be applied topically to strengthen the veins and reduce the inflammation. Witch hazel is easy to find at a local drugstore or grocer.

Gotu kola strengthens connective tissue and the integrity of the veins, helps treat current problems and leads to a reduction in the occurrence in varicose veins. It helps to reduce the excess fluid in the legs and feet as well, which is often seen with varicose veins. Typical dose is 20 drops of a 1:5 tincture up to twice a day.

Bilberry, the relative of our blueberry that is so effective with eye health, works by strengthening the connective tissues in the body, so these effects also benefit and prevent varicose veins from forming in the body. While bilberry extract is quite pricey, blueberries, grapes and blackberries can be added to the diet to take advantage of these benefits.

Warts

What is it? Warts are a common skin condition among young children. They are caused by a virus, and can be contagious when the skin is damaged by a cut or scrape. Contrary to the popular belief, they are confined to the epidermis and do not have roots but a smooth underside. Most experts believe the susceptibility to wart is determined by the individual's immune system's ability to fight off the virus when it comes in contact with it. Those with diminished immune function tend to have warts that last much longer.

Prevention: Considering that warts are contagious and most likely to be infected when cuts and scrapes are present, we can be vigilant about keeping our children's hands clean, especially when injuries are present. Yet, considering how difficult this concept is in practice, given the playful, somewhat messy nature of children, we might be more productive focusing our attention on the condition of the immune system. Ensuring limited sugar intake, plenty of beneficial whole foods and additional immune support when appropriate will help the body fight off the virus when exposed.

Additionally, a whole foods multivitamin plays a crucial role in preventing nutrient deficiencies in children, especially those with picky palates. My favorite brands are New Chapter Organics and Nordic Naturals.

Treatments: Immune support plays a major role in the treatment of warts. Astragalus root and elderberry are both child safe supplements that can be added to the daily routine while warts are present.

Garlic oil also offers valuable antiviral properties and one study shows a 100% effectiveness rate when topical garlic extract was applied directly to the affected areas, but the results took as long as 8 weeks in some individuals. I prefer to apply the oil when the children are in bed, asleep as it prevents them from walking around smelling like an Italian restaurant all day!

Zinc also offers some benefit at treating and preventing warts, so reviewing the diet and daily multivitamin to ensure plenty of zinc intake would be recommended.

Wrinkles

What is it? Wrinkles are a unique sign of age and experience. They are also seldom desired, which is why they often find themselves listed among physical conditions in need of a cure.

As we age, especially if we are often exposed to sunburn or cigarette smoke, our skin experiences oxidative damage. This literally causes us to lose the elasticity in our skin, which reduces the plump supple look our faces tend to have during our youthful days. When this elasticity is lost, and moisture is lost, lines form, especially around the eyes and mouth.

Prevention: As many other things in life, prevention really is the best medicine for wrinkles. Healthy diets and active lifestyles with plenty of hydration ensure that the skin has plenty of nutrients to remain soft and supple as long as it will.

A good whole foods based multivitamin, such as the Every Man's / Woman's One Daily by New Chapter Organics helps to ensure that plenty of nutrients are taken in on a daily basis.

A balanced approach to sun exposure also helps to prevent wrinkles. While sunlight is a healthy part of our lifestyles, too much can cause premature aging.

Treatments: Many creams and other potions marketed as reducing wrinkles actually contain ingredients that contribute to premature aging, which is quite the side effect for such a beauty treatment. There are plenty of skin care products that do help reduce the appearance of fine lines and wrinkles, but these actions are seldom found in conventional products.

Squalene provides elasticity and is naturally occurring to the skin, but begins to deplete itself during our mid-to-late twenties, resulting in the beginning of aging for many individuals. Many facial serums contain (sometimes exclusively) squalene to replace this loss. There serums moisturize the skin, without making it oily or greasy, and actually reduce the appearance of fine lines, in addition to preventing them from occurring. Squalene is derived from olives, so olive squalene is another name for the substance.

The essential oil helichrysum also helps to reduce fine lines and treats scarring, making it effective at both eliminating facial wrinkles, as well as those elsewhere on the body caused by old stretch marks form pregnancy or weight gain. It is a pricey oil, and should never be applied directly to the skin. My favorite way to take advantage of these properties is to add 10-12 drops of oil to 1/2 ounce of squalene and keep it in a dropper bottle with my cosmetics.

Rosemary is actually such a powerful antioxidant that is able to both prevent and treat wrinkles. The best way to take advantage of these benefits is topical application of a rosemary tea that can be made with 1 teaspoon of rosemary straight out of the spice cabinet steeped into 2-3 ounces of hot water.

Bilberry increases connective tissue in the body and is well known as an effective anti-aging herb. Intake of the extract is beneficial, but the related berries and fruits are just as effective. One of my favorite ways to take advantage of antioxidant rich berries is in this simple morning smoothie.

Antioxidant Berry Smoothie
2 cups frozen berry assortment (I use blueberries, blackberries and raspberries, but strawberries and even grapes are great additions as well.)
2 bananas
1 cup orange juice
Toss everything into a blender and whir until smooth.

Yeast Infections

What is it? Vaginal yeast infections are fungal infections that cause inflammation, burning and itching in the vaginal area. Many estimate that half of all visits to the gynecologist are for treatment of vaginal infections. Contrary to popular thought, however, yeast infections are not restricted to women. Men can also be infected and, while they rarely exhibit any symptoms, can pass the infection back to their spouse over and over again. Anytime I see a client with reoccurring infections, my first recommendation is to consider treating the husband.

Yeast infections are more common recently than they were in previous years because many of our common pharmaceuticals and habits encourage fungal overgrowth in the body. Antibiotics and birth control pills are two very common causes.

Prevention: The best prevention measure is to limit the use of pharmaceuticals to use when absolutely necessary. Natural birth control methods are just as effective, when used correctly and do not have the harsh side effects on the female body. Antibiotics should be limited in use not only to prevent infection, but to prevent antibiotic resistant bacteria and the many other problems we are facing because of our antibiotic addiction.

Treatments: Echinacea has been shown to reduce the reoccurrence rates in women with repeated infections. It is taken internally in conjunction with a topical or vaginal antifungal treatment for ideal results. It is effective at stimulating the immune system to fight off fungal infections, so it literally works from the inside out.

There is a popular and effective treatment that involves the placement of a garlic bulb, wrapped in gauze directly into the vagina for the night, then removing in the morning. While the treatment is certainly an effective option, I personally would not advocate placing a strong substance like garlic in such a sensitive area. Many women report burning, especially when the clove is not wrapped well enough in the gauze. Instead of attempting such a delicate task, why not take the herb orally? Garlic is just as effective when taken as a heavy addition to the diet or odorless garlic substance, and is much less risky. It is also only one of many options, which is yet another reason I simply cannot recommend resorting to such a measure.

Pau d'arco (also called teehebo) is an effective remedy that is a reliable treatment for yeast infections in both the mouth and vagina. In studies, its antifungal actions are as effective as many prescription medications, and the capsules can be taken internally. Generally, 2-3 capsules a day are sufficient, although there is not an acceptable dose for pregnant women. During pregnancy, an alternative treatment should be used.

Myrrh essential oil is highly antifungal, and effective as a topical treatment for those situations that require treatment both internally and externally. Of course, the oil cannot be applied directly to the skin undiluted, and again, it is important to consider how sensitive this particular area is when we prepare our remedies. Generally speaking, 2-3 drops of myrrh oil can be combined with 2 teaspoons of olive oil for topical application. Myrrh is not to be taken internally.

Goldenseal and Oregon grape root are also beneficial at balancing the flora, which includes bacteria and yeasts, and can keep an infection at bay. This is also to be taken internally by the non-expecting wife.

As mentioned above, the husband usually also requires treatment when the wife is experiencing recurring infections. This can be accomplished by soaking the area in an herbal bath of 1 teaspoon goldenseal powder and 1 tea spoon myrrh powder mixed with 2 cups of warm water for 10-15 minutes daily. This should be combined with oral intake of pau d'arco and garlic for 10-14 days to prevent re-infection.

Probiotics are essential for any fungal overgrowth situation, whether oral or vaginal and in both men and women. These are taken orally, and should be used as both a preventative measure and a treatment.

Section Three: Botanical Apothecary

Arnica
(*Arnica montana*)

Arnica is an ancient flowering herb found wild in many mountainous regions of Europe. It has a long history as a medical herb, and this two foot tall plant has been used successfully throughout history for many of the same reasons we enjoy it today. Modern day use is common among both homeopaths and herbalists, which account for most of the herb's sales. It is generally used topically for aches and sprains, especially sports injuries.

When to use it: Arnica relieves pain and inflammation, soothing sore muscles in the body. These properties are especially useful after increased physical activity or sports. It is ideal for bruises, sprains, and other inflammation of the skin.

Culinary Medicine: Since arnica is not an herb we take internally, we do not blend it with our meals.

Optimal Dose: Oils and ointments should contain 10-15% arnica.

When to avoid it: Arnica is not to be applied to broken skin. Some individuals with extremely sensitive skin or conditions such as eczema may experience a rash like reaction to the herb. In these cases, use should be discontinued.

Astragalus
(*Astragalus membranaceus*)

This Chinese legume has been used for centuries as an immune support and treatment for cancer. More recently, it has become popular for its adaptogenic properties, which help the body adapt to stress and other environmental changes. It is often used for infections, especially those in the respiratory and urinary tract.

It is also often combined with ginseng to prevent winter bugs, which follows the accepted belief that it is most effective against viral illness.

Research shows that it helps reduce the frequency and intensity of the common cold.

It is clinically shown to increase the number of white blood cells, which are our fighter cells when the body is facing illness. It is also beneficial for cancer patients, as it helps to return the T-cells back to near normal function.

When to use it: Astragalus is a great preventative herb, and can be taken prior to the onset of illness. In the Hawkins' home, astragalus is taken prior to amusement park visits, plane flights, holiday parties and even large play groups. In glycerite form, it can be added to a morning glass of juice for ease of administration.

Culinary Medicine: As a legume, there are many recipes for astragalus soup or other warming meals. It is not readily available in most regions, however, so is taken as a supplement.

Optimal Dose: Astragalus can be taken three times a day in a tincture or glycerite with a 1:5 ratio. Ideal dose for an adult is 15-30 drops of extract, each administration.

When to avoid it: Astragalus is safe for most situations, even with long term use. There are no known contraindications, which means that there are no known situations that should exclude use of the herb.

Basil
(*Ocimum basilicum*)

This bushy plant has been cultivated for millennia and is native to Asia's tropical regions and the Mediterranean. The name comes from a Greek word meaning "royal", and the plant has been esteemed as a regal plant throughout history.

Basil is rich in antioxidants, which may be a contributing factor to the common use of one type of basil, holy basil as an adaptogen. Even the scent of basil is known to be uplifting, bringing about mental clarity.

It is also anti-inflammatory, which makes it beneficial for depression, headaches and even some digestive disorders and helps to regulate the intestinal flora, another great benefit to this with digestive disorders.

When to use it: Basil is the "go to" herb for times of intense stress or major routine changes such as a vacation or move. It helps the body adapt to change well and supports the immune system.

To take advantage of its digestive benefits, basil can play a starring role in many of our standard dishes. As the foods are being prepared, the scent is released, providing emotional and mental benefits, and the regular consumption during mealtime is plenty to enjoy the digestive benefits.

Culinary Medicine: Basil blends well with just about any dish, but pasta and chicken seem to be the most popular. The green pesto sauce features large amounts of basil and is a very versatile sauce.

Basil Pesto
4 cups fresh basil leaves
1 cup grated Parmesan cheese
1/2 cup olive oil
3/4 cup pine nuts
3 T minced garlic
salt and pepper to taste
In a blender or food processor, chop the nuts and basil. Add the garlic and blend. Open the top and slowly add the oil. Finish with the cheese and spices. This makes enough to use now and freeze half for later. Toss 1 cup with 1 pound cooked pasta, scoop it over grilled chicken or spread over cream cheese for a party dip. The uses are limitless!

Optimal Dose: Basil is best enjoyed as a culinary herb, but when dosing with the holy basil for added benefits, the typical dose is 800 mg dried herb per day.

When to avoid it: Pregnant women should limit their use of the herb to culinary purposes.

Bilberry
(*Vaccinium myrtillus*)

Bilberry, also called huckleberry, is a relative of our common blueberry plant, and even grows on small shrubs, not unlike the blueberry. It is native to Europe, and has been used for over a thousand years in herbal medicine as a treatment for dysentery. Internally, it helps to treat childhood diarrhea, but is perhaps better known for its effects on the adult population.

Modern day use of bilberry focuses on its use as an anti-aging supplement. A compound called anthocyanidins, which are found in abundance it bilberry and many of its relatives, has been shown to improve night vision and overall vision that has been damaged as a result of diabetes or age related macular degeneration. It also helps soothe minor throat irritations.

When to use it: Bilberry is useful for children experiencing diarrhea, and for adults with diabetes or macular degeneration. For both uses, a liquid extract, whether tincture or glycerite, is ideal for ease of administration.

Culinary Medicine: While bilberries are not readily available for consumption, its relatives, the blueberry and grape, are easy to find any many markets. Both of these foods contain the same dark pigment that is responsible for many of the health benefits found in the bilberry and can easily be added liberally to the diet to obtain these benefits. Blueberry smoothies are a great morning treat, and grapes, when frozen, provide a soothing summertime treat for a sore throat.

Optimal Dose: 5-10 grams of crushed fruit or equivalent daily

When to avoid it: Bilberry is generally considered to be safe, and there are no known situations that would require avoidance of the herb.

Burdock
(*Arctium lappa*)

Burdock is a common weed, and like many common weeds, contains powerful detoxification abilities. It also contains many minerals, which are beneficial during detoxification, since they are often lost during the elimination process.

Another benefit of the herb is it can help to regulate the intestinal flora, which is often disturbed by the intake of many common pharmaceuticals and lifestyle habits.

When to use it: Burdock is beneficial during bouts of eczema flare ups, constipation or sluggish bowels and as a detoxification boost.

Culinary Medicine: Burdock is generally consumed as an herbal tea, not an addition to the solid diet.

Optimal Dose: Tea made with 2.5 grams of the herb per one cup of water can be consumed 2-3 times per day.

When to avoid it: Burdock is generally considered to be safe, and there are no known situations that would require avoidance of the herb.

Calendula
(*Calendula officinalis*)

This bright yellow flowering herb is also known as marigold, although other species also go by the common name marigold, which is why we often rely on the botanical names of a plant. Pot marigold and garden marigold are two other common names for the herb.

Calendula is native to the Egyptian and Mediterranean regions and was a commonly used plant in ancient Roman and Grecian medicine. As a medicinal plant, it is prized for its anti-inflammatory properties and ability to stimulate wound healing.

In addition to its use as an herbal remedy, it also provides a reliable bright yellow dye for clothing.

When to use it: Calendula is handy herb to have in the home, as its uses are practically endless. During a common childhood ear infection, the addition of calendula to the garlic oil treatment can bring soothing relief from the inflammation. The assistance in wound healing is valuable for the new mommy with a cesarean scar or sore perineum, and can treat countless other minor scrapes and injuries. Likewise, the soothing herb brings relief to irritated skin when conditions such as eczema are present.

Culinary Medicine: Calendula is generally applied topically, so it is not combined with our meal preparations.

Optimal Dose: Calendula containing creams should provide at least 5% herb content. Calendula can be found in many ointments, balms, salves, creams and even oils. These preparations are fun and easy to make at home, as long as the correct type of marigold has been obtained and identified.

When to avoid it: There are not any conditions that prohibit the use of calendula, although it should be discontinued if allergic symptoms are observed.

Cascara Sagreda
(*Rhamnus purshiana*)

Cascara is a tree native to the Western regions of North America. For herbal use, the bark of the tree is harvested, dried, and aged for at least one year, to prevent causing harsh intestinal irritation.

The bark is then used to treat constipation, and is gentle enough to use even when hemorrhoids or anal fissures are present.

The name comes from the early Spanish terms meaning sacred and bark, which demonstrates how prized the herb was to the early native culture.

When to use it: Cascara is useful for constipation of any kind, but is generally best as a last resort for children, after other nutritional and dietary remedies have been attempted. Results are generally seen in under eight hours.

Culinary Medicine: Cascara is not an herb well suited for dietary consumption, but other fiber rich foods or herbs with very mild laxatives could be added to the diet regularly to prevent the need for stronger remedies such as cascara.

Optimal Dose: Cascara is taken on an "as needed" basis, so the correct dose is the absolute minimum amount necessary to produce a bowel movement. It should never be taken longer than a week or two without direct supervision from the family physician.

It should also be taken into consideration that laxatives will often take a few hours to bring about desired effects. So, additional intake should be avoided until ample time has passed to determine the dose to be insufficient.

When to avoid it: It should not be taken when licorice root or corticosteroids are also in the routine, and any laxative is to be avoided when there is a blockage or other intestinal problem that would prohibit the use of a laxative. These can include but are not limited to irritable bowel syndrome, Chron's disease, appendicitis, and even abdominal pain without a known source. If in doubt, contact the family physician for guidance.

Chamomile
(*Matricaria recutita*)

Chamomile is the ancient romantic herb, with a sweet, apple like scent. It is native to parts of both Europe and Asia and is perhaps one of the most important medicinal plants we harvest. The name chamomile comes from Greek words literally meaning ground apple, which is appropriate considering how closely the scent of chamomile's yellow flowers resemble that of a sweet apple.

Medicinal values include mild sedative properties, which most individuals associate with the plant, but herbalists tend to place a greater value on its anti-inflammatory properties.

When to use it: The most common use of chamomile is as a digestive aid. It improves digestion that may be hindered by multiple reasons, including improper intestinal flora, stress during consumption and minor gastric upsets. When brewed into a tea, it offers gentle relief, and can combat inflammation as well. These digestive benefits extend to the youngest members of our family, as chamomile is an effective and reliable remedy for colic.

It is also useful topically as a soothing treatment for inflammatory conditions. It is especially suitable for infants and children during problems such as diaper rash because it is extremely mild and gentle, yet effective. The herb has the ability to penetrate deeply into the skin, bringing about healing from the deepest layers. Likewise, the herb is also beneficial for assisting in the healing of wounds.

Chamomile tea is generally understood to bring about restfulness and prepare the individual for a good night's sleep. This benefit is also found in the essential oil through aromatherapy.

Culinary Medicine: Chamomile tea is a great tasting drink for all ages to enjoy. Children that tend to have a sweet tooth can blend the tea with apple or white grape juice for a more pleasant tasting remedy, ideally suited for hectic holidays and birthdays.

Optimal Dose: Chamomile is often taken in preparations made with up to 1/4 cup of dried flowering tops. Warm baths can also benefit from including a tea bag or ball with up to a cup of the dried herb.

When to avoid it: Those with allergies to the ragweed family may also have a chamomile allergy, otherwise, the herb is gentle enough to be enjoyed by anyone.

Chaste berry
(*Agni casti fructus*)

Chaste berry, also known as chaste tree fruit or vitex is an herb used throughout history to directly affect the hormones. It is a small shrub, native to Greece and Italy. Historic use included consumption by monks and women with soldier husbands off to battle, as it was thought to reduce libido, ensuring the celibacy necessary to such individuals or circumstances.

Modern research does not back these specific uses, but does confirm its use as a female tonic, helping to regulate the hormones. It decreases the production of prolactin, which is responsible for milk production and helps to correct luteal phase defects and relieve PMS.

When to use it: Vitex is ideally suited for use among women with irregular menstrual cycles and heavy PMS. It is not ideally suited for those trying to conceive unless there is difficulty based on luteal phase defects. Once pregnancy is achieved, the herb should be discontinued slowly with the aid of a midwife or wholistic professional.

Culinary Medicine: Vitex is not to be taken in excess and is best taken as a liquid extract, so culinary intake is not common.

Optimal Dose: In a tincture with a 1:5 ratio, ideal dosage is 0.15-0.2ml per day.

When to avoid it: Vitex should be avoided during pregnancy and breastfeeding. It can inhibit the production of milk in the body.

Chickweed
(*Stellaria media*)

Chickweed, true to its name, is a common weed, readily available worldwide. It is safe for consumption, and offers an abundance of rich minerals that benefit the body during detoxification. Yet, it is most useful to the herbalist for its external benefits, including the anti-inflammatory effects and the ability to increase the permeability of bacterial cell walls and draw out toxins.

When to use it: It is best suited for topical application to wounds, rashes and infections, but can also be added to herbal extract blends to increase the absorption of other compounds and restore the nutrient stores of the body.

Culinary Medicine: Chickweed is not generally used as a culinary herb.

Optimal Dose: Chickweed is best in a topical preparation containing at least 10%-15% of the herb. For internal use, exact dosing will depend heavily on the other herbs in the blend.

When to avoid it: Chickweed is generally considered to be safe, and there are no known situations that would require avoidance of the herb.

Dandelion
(*Taraxacom officinale*)

Dandelions are more than a common lawn weed, in herbal medicine, they are extremely beneficial and even prized for their contributions to overall health. This beneficial weed has been used as a medicinal plant for over a thousand years, and is best known for its ability to support liver function and reduce the severity of various skin conditions, including eczema.

Dandelions also help to regulate the intestinal flora, which is another essential benefit of any detoxification routine, as do the numerous minerals available in the herb.

When to use it: Dandelion extract is ideally suited for those with inflammatory skin conditions or other forms of dermatitis. It is also a beneficial herbal bitter, which means that it can stimulate appetite and assist the digestive process.

Culinary Medicine: Dandelions are a fantastic addition to a garden salad. They add a bit of bright color to the overall appearance, and the flavor blends well with any combination of greens. However, it is important to note that consumption of dandelions should not include any wild harvested varieties. Considering the common use of herbicides used in today's lawn care, most dandelions are laden with toxins and not suitable for human consumption. Instead, opt for dandelions that have been grown specifically for dietary use.

Optimal Dose: In the diet, dandelions can be added liberally to a salad or other green food. As an extract, ideal dose is 10-15 drops of a 1:5 ratio tincture up to 3 times per day.

When to avoid it: Dandelion should not be taken internally when gall stones are present or when there is an obstruction of the bile ducts without first consulting with a professional for assistance.

Dong quai
(*Angelica sinensis*)

This Chinese herb is second only to licorice in use, yet many in the United States have never heard of it. Merck first introduced it in 1899 under the trade name Eumenol, which was marketed as a female tonic.

Dong quai is pronounced "tang kwai", and the herb is well suited for regulating the female reproductive system, encouraging childbearing. It is especially beneficial for balancing black cohosh, as the two work in a synergesic manner.

When to use it: Dong quai is perfect for assorted female complaints, such as hormone regulation, PMS and irregular cycles. It is ideally taken in a liquid extract, such as a tincture of glycerite.

Culinary Medicine: Dong quai is not an herb typically suited for dietary consumption.

Optimal Dose: Ideal dose for dong quai is 2-4 g of the dried root total per day. This can be taken in the liquid equivalent, spread through 2-3 doses.

When to avoid it: Dong quai should not be taken during pregnancy or by anyone that may become pregnant. While it is well suited to prepare the body for childbirth, it should not be taken once the body has become more regular and is ready to achieve childbirth.

Echinacea
(*Echinacea purpurea*)

Also known as purple coneflower, echinacea has spent quite a bit of time as the top selling herb in the country. Considering our annual expenses in over the counter cold remedies, this is not surprising. Echinacea, as suspected is highly effective at treating colds, reducing the duration by an average of 30%. It is also effective at treating upper respiratory infections and yeast or fungal overgrowth, including vaginal yeast infections.

Contrary to popular belief, echinacea is not well suited to function as an effective preventative herb, and research shows very little effect at preventing viral infections. However, when begun at the very first sign of infection, the herb can effectively prevent the illness from developing into a full blown cold, instead the symptoms were less severe and full recovery was much faster.

In treatment of vaginal yeast infection, the herb also offers the benefit of a reduced re-occurrence rate, which is significant considering the typically high rate of re-occurrence with this type of infection.

Children also benefit from the effectiveness of the herb, as studies show that intake of echinacea during an ear infection leads to a much lower re-occurrence rate. Childhood ear infections are yet another illness prone to re-occurrence with conventional medications.

When to use it: Echinacea is suitable for nearly every viral infection, including all of our winter bugs, and respiratory infections. It should be taken at the first sign of infection and continued throughout the course of the illness. As a single extract, it can be combined with other herbal remedies that are suited to the specific symptoms of the infection, offering added benefits.

When an ear infection is present, the herb can be beneficial in both an ear oil preparation and as an internal immune stimulant. As with a respiratory infection, the herb should be continued throughout the duration of the infection until all symptoms have cleared.

For yeast infections or other chronic fungal overgrowth, echinacea is suitable for internal treatment to boost immunity and regulate the balance of yeasts and bacteria in the body (also known as the flora).

Culinary Medicine: Echinacea is generally taken as an extract, either tincture or glycerite, so dietary use is not common.

Optimal Dose: Five ml of a liquid extract can be taken three to five times a day. A tincture should be prepared in a 1:5 ratio.

When to avoid it: Echinacea should not be taken on a long term basis. Generally, eight weeks is the maximum time frame for daily intake, with a minimum break from the herb of two to three weeks before beginning treatment again. However, when we consider that the plant should not be taken on a preventative basis, rather a treatment option, it is difficult to imagine a situation that would require the long term use of the herb.

Additionally, the herb is said to be contraindicated (ie: not suitable for) those with autoimmune disorders or those with progressive disorders, such as tuberculosis.

Elderberry
(*Sambucus nigra*)

The elder plant, both the flowers and berries have been used medicinally since the time of Hippocrates. It was traditionally used as a remedy for the flu and common cold, and today, that tradition remains strong, as many natural cold and flu preparations still contain parts of the elder plant.

Dr. Shook, an herbal pioneer discussed the herb many times in his work, and fervently believed that the common cold and flu could be cured worldwide by the use of a blend containing elder and peppermint with yarrow.

The berries are also frequently made into a syrup preparation and are thus suitable as an immune booster, working to prevent viral infections during times of increased exposure.

When to use it: Elder is ideally suited for use as an immune stimulant and as a remedy for viral infections, particularly the flu and common cold. Elderberry syrup is a staple in the Hawkins' home during the fall and winter months. When additional remedies are also useful, elderberry can be continued throughout the illness, as it blends readily with many other herbs.

Culinary Medicine: Elderberry jam is a common addition to many breakfast tables in some countries. While it is not as commonly available in the United States, some gourmet grocers carry foods featuring elderberries. The berries must be cook, however, since the raw plant contains a cyanide producing substance that is inactivated by cooking.

Optimal Dose: 1-3 tablespoons syrup a day

When to avoid it: Elder berries and flowers are generally considered to be safe, and there are no known situations that would require avoidance of the herb.

Eyebright
(*Euphrasia officinalis*)

As one can imagine, this herb is ideally suited to benefit one particular part of the body, the eyes. It brings about speedy and effective recovery for many common problems the eyes may face, including both pink eye and styes.

When to use it: We turn to eyebright anytime we have an eye infection that requires treatment. Liquid extracts are ideal for ease of administration. A warm, damp washcloth with about 2-3 drops of the herb applied directly to the affected area can be left in place up to 5 minutes or until it becomes uncomfortable. This can be repeated 3-5 times a day until relief is seen.

Culinary Medicine: We do not typically consume this herb, so it is not well suited for culinary purposes.

Optimal Dose: Eyebright is typically applied topically as a compress, not taken internally, as it has a fairly low toxicity level. Unless consulting with a professional, it is best to avoid ingesting eyebright.

When to avoid it: Eyebright is generally considered to be safe, but should be avoided by those that are pregnant or breastfeeding and should only be applied externally.

Fenugreek
(*Trigonella foenum-graecum*)

This ancient herb is native to the Mediterranean region and has been used medicinally since the ancient Egyptians, as an herb to induce childbirth. Throughout history, it was popular for many different female complaints, and is still a valuable herb today.

Fenugreek is perhaps best known for its ability to increase milk production, but also has many additional properties that should be taken into consideration as well. It is effective at reducing cholesterol levels, reducing blood sugar levels, and externally as an anti-inflammatory compress.

When to use it: Fenugreek is the herb of choice for many lactation consultants, but it is important to keep in mind the potential for lowering blood sugar will also make its way to the baby. When other remedies have not done the job, it can offer valuable benefits to the milk supply, but the possible effects on the baby should be kept in mind. The herb, whether taken in tea form of liquid extract, can cause a mild maple syrup scent to the milk, but this is harmless.

It is ideally suited for diabetics and others with tendencies towards high blood sugar (prediabetics) or those with high cholesterol without hypoglycemia.

Culinary Medicine: Fenugreek is typically consumed as an herbal tea and is well suited for blending with many other medicinal herbs.

Optimal Dose: In a 1:5 tincture, daily dose is 30 ml. This can be broken into three doses of 10 ml.

When to avoid it: Fenugreek should be avoided by those with hypoglycemia and should not be taken during pregnancy.

Garlic
(*Allium sativum*)

Garlic has been the subject of thousands of scientific studies, as its medicinal uses are numerous. Garlic reduces cholesterol levels, bringing the ratios back into a healthy range. It also helps lower blood pressure, which is significant because the two often occur together in an individual.

In the diet, garlic is also shown to play a powerful role in the prevention of multiple types of cancer. Many trials also show these benefits from an odorless garlic supplement, but fresh dietary herbs are always the ideal treatment.

When to use it: Garlic is the herb of choice for those with high cholesterol or blood pressure. It can be added liberally to the diet to obtain these benefits, and successfully treats both conditions.

Garlic is also useful for boosting the immune response and fighting / treating infections of all kinds. The best way to take advantage of these benefits is to increase the consumption of garlic during times of illness or increased exposure to illness.

Culinary Medicine: Obviously culinary medicine is the ideal way to consume the herb. Garlic is a staple in many pasta dishes, salad dressings, flavored breads and chicken dishes. It adds a special kick to the plate, bringing with it plenty of flavor.

Garlic Bread
2 cloves garlic
1 stick butter (melted)
1 tablespoon parsley
Mince the garlic, allow to sit, exposed to the air for 10 –12 minutes, then add to the butter and parsley. Baste generously onto a sliced baguette, making sure the garlic is spread evenly along the loaf. Brown in the oven at 400 degrees for 5-8 minutes or until the bread is slightly toasted. Slice and serve hot!

Optimal Dose: Standard dose of garlic is 4g a day

When to avoid it: Garlic has slight blood thinning properties, so those taking or avoiding blood thinners should consult a physician prior to taking medicinal amounts of garlic. Dietary amounts are generally suitable for everyone.

Gingko
(*Gingko biloba*)

Gingko is one of our most ancient trees, with a rich medicinal tradition to match. It has been used in Europe and Asia for millennia, primarily for its ability to improve circulation in the elderly and improve mental stamina in the general population.

Other traditional uses include respiratory infection, male erectile dysfunction and altitude sickness.

When to use it: Gingko is well suited for individual with Alzheimer's, but can also benefit anyone that could use an increase in mental clarity, cognitive function and enhanced memory, which is just about everyone!

Culinary Medicine: Gingko is one herb that is best used as a standardized preparation, so it is unsuitable for culinary use.

Optimal Dose: Gingko should be standardized to contain 24% gingko-flavone glycosides and 6% terpene lactones. The dose is 120-240 mg daily, divided into three doses.

When to avoid it: Those with cardiac disorders should consult a physician prior to use. Additionally, gingko has mild blood thinning properties, so those taking or avoiding blood thinners should consult with a professional to determine if gingko is a suitable supplement for their routine.

Hawthorne leaf
(*Crataegus oxycantha*)

Hawthorne is an herb that has been studies in depth in some European countries, and many different parts of the plant have been used medicinally, including the leaf, flower and berries. The herb has a long traditional use as a cardiotonic, and was a favorite among the ancient Greeks.

The plant is known to dilate the arteries, leading to a decrease in blood pressure and improved blood supply, which forms the basis for its primary use throughout the world today.

When to use it: Hawthorne is suitable for just about any cardiac condition. It improved overall heart function and has even been used to treat angina. For use in treating hypertension (high blood pressure), results often take up to 6 months to be fully evident, so patience should be exercised when treating with hawthorne, but trials show these benefits are equal to that of pharmaceutical hypertension medications, without the dangerous side effects.

Culinary Medicine: Hawthorne is not typically used as a culinary herb.

Optimal Dose: Dose varies greatly depending on the potency and the brand, but standardized extracts of 160-900 mg a day divided into three doses are typical.

When to avoid it: Hawthorne is generally considered to be safe, and there are no known situations that would require avoidance of the herb.

Kava Kava
(*Piper methysticum*)

Kava, native to the South Pacific islands, is prized by traditional communities for its relaxing effect on the body. Many ceremonies consist of a ritual drink of a kava tea or beverage, and guests are honored with native tea blends as a sign of welcome.

These uses lead to the reputation kava holds as an anti-anxiety drug. If taken in excess, however, the herb can cause symptoms of inebriation.

When to use it: Kava is a great tension reliever for stressful situations, holiday gatherings and even family vacations. It is well suited for nervous anxiety and restlessness, but is generally an adult remedy.

Culinary Medicine: Aside from the native tea, Kava is not generally taken as a food, rather a medicinal drink or supplement.

Optimal Dose: As an herbal tea, 1-2 teaspoons of kava are steeped into an eight ounce glass of water. It should not be taken daily for longer than three months.

When to avoid it: Pregnant and breastfeeding women should not take kava. Those that are taking other drugs that affect the central nervous system, such as alcohol or barbiturates should also avoid kava, as the herb can intensify the effects of such drugs. Finally, no individual should drive a vehicle of operate machinery after taking kava, as it may cause a feeling of inebriation.

Lavender
(*Lavendula augustifolia*)

These native Mediterranean herbs are named from a Latin word meaning "to wash" which brings to remembrance the ancient Roman bath houses and modern aromatherapy spas. There are over 28 varieties of this herb, which can be useful from everything from scenting bed linens to gracing the tables of fine restaurants.

Medicinally, lavender produces an essential oil that offers many beneficial properties, including treating insomnia, intestinal problems and even mood disturbances.

It also offers potent antibacterial properties, and has been used to treat wounds, infections and as a hospital disinfectant.

When to use it: Lavender is well suited for restlessness and irritability. For these treatments, an essential oil blend diffused throughout the room is a great way to enjoy the herb and its benefits.

As an antiseptic, lavender oil is the ideal form of treatment, and is one of the only essential oils that can actually be applied to the skin undiluted, although it is still ideal to dilute with carrier oil in a 1:1 ratio.

When added to the diet, lavender also helps improve digestive function, providing the same soothing benefits to the stomach that it brings to the mind through external use.

Culinary Medicine: Lavender is a gourmet kitchen herb, as blends well with any other Mediterranean herbs at the table. One popular way to incorporate the herb into mealtime is by the addition of an Herbs de Provence blend. These herbs can be kept in the spice cabinet and tossed onto roasted chicken, fish or most vegetables. They are wonderful over a pile of roasted red potatoes with a drizzle of olive oil and a dash of sea salt.

Herbs de Provence Spice Blend
2 tablespoons lavender buds
1 tablespoon basil

1 tablespoon oregano
1 tablespoon thyme
1 tablespoon rosemary

Optimal Dose: Lavender tea is typically brewed with 1-2 teaspoons of the herb per 8 ounce glass of water.

When to avoid it: Lavender is generally considered to be safe, and there are no known situations that would require avoidance of the herb.

Lemon balm
(*Melissa officinalis*)

Like many of our most prized medicinal herbs, lemon balm is native to the eastern Mediterranean and western Asian regions. It is a part of the mint family, but contains a lemon like scent, hence the name. This small shrub is also the source of a valuable essential oil with potent antiviral properties.

A traditional treatment of lemon balm involved steeping the herb in wine for topical application of surgical sites and wounds. Modern uses, however focus on the internal benefits to the digestive system and nervous system.

When to use it: Lemon balm is well suited for nervous restlessness, and for digestive disorders, which often appear together. It is a rich source of powerful antioxidants, and contributes to overall health when stress or other factors are causing irritability or tension.

Culinary Medicine: Lemon balm is not often taken as a culinary herb, rather as a tea or within a blend of herbs for tea.

Optimal Dose: For an herbal tea, 2-4 g of herb are steeped into 8 ounces of water.

When to avoid it: Lemon balm is generally considered to be safe, and there are no known situations that would require avoidance of the herb.

Licorice
(*Glycyrrhiza glabra*)

Licorice is so much more than the flavoring for chewy childhood candies. It is a perennial herb native to the Mediterranean region and one of the most researched herbs in medicine. First documented in Egyptian medicinal records and Assyrian clay tablets, licorice has been used throughout history for colds, the flu and other viral infections.

While it remains a valuable herb in botanical medicine, it contains a substance called glycyrrhizin, which can lead to cardiac problems. However modern supplements generally remove this compound, and the resulting product (called deglycyrrhizinated licorice) can be taken for equally effective results without the concern regarding the safety of the medication.

Other uses for the herb include topical treatments of skin conditions such as eczema, internal treatment for gastric ulcers, and chronic fungal conditions.

When to use it: Licorice is often added to cough and cold herbal blends, and is a reliable treatment for respiratory concerns. Bronchitis, coughs and viral infections all benefit from the use of licorice in an antiviral blend.

When dealing with eczema, the topical application of an extract has been shown to reduce the need for corticosteroids.

For gastric ulcers and fungal conditions, it is important to purchase standardized deglycyrrhizinated licorice extracts for optimum benefit and reduced risk.

Culinary Medicine: Licorice is a common flavoring agent for candies, but the active properties are not available in candy form.

Optimal Dose: 15 ml up to 4 times a day for six to eight weeks

When to avoid it: There are many individuals that should not take licorice as an herbal supplement. Pregnant and breastfeeding women should avoid the herb, as should anyone with a liver condition of any kind. Those with kidney disorders, cardiac disorders or low potassium levels should also void use of licorice. Individuals taking hormonal therapies should consult with a professional prior to taking licorice as it can interact under certain circumstances.

Marshmallow
(Althea officinalis)

Marshmallow is a perennial herb from the Mediterranean region that contains thick mucilage, which forms a gel like substance when mixed with water. It has been a staple of herbal medicine for over two thousand years, dating back to at least the 9th century BC. The traditional uses also focused on the thick mucilage, which soothes inflammation when applied topically.

When to use it: Marshmallow is ideal for any respiratory condition that leads to a sore throat or cough. The gel like substance soothes the irritation, promoting clearer breathing and reducing pain caused by the inflammation. This also helps to reduce the coughing spells, and has become a common ingredient in cough syrups for these benefits.

Culinary Medicine: Marshmallow is not typically consumed as a culinary herb.

Optimal Dose: In a tincture with the typical 1:5 ratio, up to 10-25 ml can be given per dose, and dosing can occur up to three times a day. As a syrup, the dose would be 10 ml, to soothe throat irritation.

When to avoid it: Marshmallow root is generally considered to be safe, and there are no known situations that would require avoidance of the herb.

Milk thistle
(*Silybum marianum*)

Milk thistle is a tall plant that first built a reputation by preventing poisoning in mushroom toxicity cases. This has led to its importance as a poison control remedy, which would be due to its powerful actions on the liver, our detoxification organ.

Used medicinally since the times of the ancient Greeks and Romans, milk thistle is one of my absolute favorite herbs. It offers liver supportive benefits for the average individual, increasing the natural detoxification process, but is strong enough to actually help rejuvenate the liver in cases of hepatitis, alcoholic cirrhosis and exposure to harsh chemicals.

When to use it: Considering that a sluggish liver can contribute to anything from diabetes to morning sickness and even eczema, supplementation with milk thistle is beneficial for just about any health problem. Even when the illness is significant enough to require advanced measures such as pharmaceuticals, the milk thistle can help the body to process these medications effectively.

Specific situations that especially benefit from the herb include chemotherapy, alcoholism or even heavy and moderate drinking, use of pharmaceuticals or over the counter remedies, exposure to chemicals in daily environment, pregnancy and even a change in diet.

Culinary Medicine: Milk thistle is not generally consumed as a dietary herb.

Optimal Dose: Milk thistle is an herb that is well suited to standardization, since the silymarin is not well absorbed by the intestines. Ensuring that a supplement contains at least 80% silymarin helps increase the potential absorption rate of the active compound.

When to avoid it: Milk thistle is generally considered to be safe, and there are no known situations that would require avoidance of the herb. Studies show that even with daily, long term use, the benefits are not reduced and no adverse side effects have been observed.

Oregano
(Ociginum vulgare)

Oregano, native to the Mediterranean region, is a small shrub with a rich history among ancient cultures, especially Greece and Rome. It was considered to be a sign of joy and laurels of the herb adorned the heads of new brides.

The oil from the plant is the part most commonly used in herbal medicine, and has shown potent antibacterial properties that even exceed that of conventional antibiotics.

Oregano also has an extremely high antioxidant content, which increases the benefit when taken during an illness, and makes it a valuable culinary herb.

When to use it: Oregano is best taken at the first sign of an illness to fight off infection. It is particularly beneficial with stronger infections that might otherwise require pharmaceutical treatment.

Culinary Medicine: Oregano is a popular culinary herb, especially common among pizza and Italian, Greek and Spanish dishes. Consumed as a part of the diet, oregano has the potential to increase the detoxification of the body through the valuable antioxidants, and serve as preventative medicine, helping to fight off potential illness.

A great way to incorporate oregano in the diet is to keep some by the stove and toss onto pasta, chicken and vegetable dishes. Here is a great example.

Oregano Pasta
1 pound pasta, any shape
Juice and zest of one lemon
1 tablespoon rosemary
3 tablespoons oregano
1/4 cup olive oil
1/3 cup grated hard Italian cheese (such as parmesan)
1/4 cup olives
1/4 cup sun dried tomatoes

Cook pasta according to package directions. Drain and toss with oil, herbs, olives, tomatoes and lemon. Top with cheese. Serve immediately or allow to chill and serve at room temperature.

Optimal Dose: There is no standard dose for oregano, as it is an herb that has the most benefit when used in culinary purposes.

When to avoid it: Culinary use of oregano is generally considered to be safe, and there are no known situations that would require avoidance of the herb in food preparations.

Oregon grape root
(*Mahonia aquifolia)*

Oregon grape root is native to North America and, although it has a long historic use in medicine, has only recently become one of the more popular treatments. Much of this is due to the possible endangered state of the goldenseal plant, which offers many similar properties. As cautious use of goldenseal has decreased, Oregon grape root has been the substitute of choice.

The herb offers potent antibacterial properties and is safe enough for young children, in appropriate doses.

When to use it: Oregon grape root is often blended with echinacea to treat infections of all kinds. This blend is especially beneficial for the more powerful infections that do not respond well to typical immune support.

Other conditions that benefit form use of the herb include eczema, acne, ear infections, diarrhea, parasites and sinus infections.

Culinary Medicine: Oregon grape root is not well suited for culinary use, as it is typically reserved for illness, not prevention.

Optimal Dose: Oregon grape root should not be used for long term treatment, as it can lead to a decrease in Vitamin B absorption. For a standard 1:5 tincture, 1/2 to 1 teaspoon up to three times a day is the adult dose, however many blends successfully use the herb in smaller amounts combined with other supportive herbs.

When to avoid it: Diabetics, pregnant and breastfeeding women, and individuals with a history of stroke, hypertension or glaucoma should all avoid the use of Oregon grape root.

Peppermint
(*Mentha x piperita*)

This aromatic herb is found growing wild throughout Europe, but has also become a common plant in the United States for the production of peppermint oil. Mint leaves have played a role in medicine since the ancient Egyptians, and were common throughout both the Roman and the Grecian cultures.

For stomach ailments, it is often combined with chamomile to treat even the most sensitive of individuals, including children. It offers powerful antiseptic properties, especially useful in the extracted essential oil, and the menthol content helps to soothe sunburns and provide clear breathing during respiratory infections, when inhaled.

When to use it: Peppermint oil helps to relieve headaches, nausea and promotes clear breathing when inhaled, so diffusion throughout a room is the best method to achieve these effects. The oil is also very strong and should never be applied undiluted on the skin, especially the face, and is not suitable for young children, even when diluted.

Internally, it is useful for gastric upsets, including indigestion, nausea, heartburn and other similar problems. Enteric coated capsules are best for this use, as they assure that the medicinal properties make it through the digestive system.

It is also well suited to treat the common cold and viral infections. It plays a key role in the Children's Composition formula, which also contains elderflower and yarrow and is believed by many to be the absolute best remedy for these winter infections.

Culinary Medicine: For improved digestion, an after dinner mint containing real peppermint extract is an ideal way of taking advantage of the herb's best qualities.

Optimal Dose: For a standard 1:5 tincture, 10 ml can be taken up to 3 times a day.

When to avoid it: When gallstones are present, a professional should be consulted prior to use. Otherwise, there are no known problems with intake of peppermint.

Plantain
(*Plantago lanceolata*)

Plantain is widely available throughout the European and Asian regions, and has been valued medicinally since the times of the ancient Greeks and Romans.

The herb offers two valuable applications, both directly relates to its potent anti-inflammatory properties. It soothes the throat, preventing excessive coughing and when applied topically, relieves skin inflammation.

When to use it: Plantain is a useful ingredient in an herbal cough syrup. It brings both symptomatic relief through the soothing properties and helps to reduce the coughing spells.

For skin conditions such as eczema and temporary irritations, the herb is a valuable ingredient in a soothing balm or salve. Some products feature plantain exclusively, and most basic herb walks cover the topic of plucking wild plantain and applying it to common outdoors scrapes and irritations by combining the fresh herb with small amounts of water.

Culinary Medicine: Plantain is often consumed as a tea, but that is the extant of its common culinary use.

Optimal Dose: For a standard 1:5 tincture, the dose is 7 ml up to 3 times a day, but as an ingredient in cough syrups, less plantain may be used in a blend with other effective herbs. For topical applications, the herb is used in an ointment with at least a 10-15% herb content.

When to avoid it: Plantain is generally considered to be safe, and there are no known situations that would require avoidance of the herb.

Red clover
(*Trifolium pratense*)

Red clover is often grown through the world as feed for cattle, but also offers medicinal benefits for humans, especially females.

This legume is rich in phytoestrogens, which help maintain proper bone density in post menopausal women, and treat hot flashes and night sweats. Many experts suggest caution with red clover and other herbs containing phytoestrgens, based on the problematic effects of estrogens in the body, especially related to breast and other hormonal cancers. Research, however, has not found phytoestrogens to have the same effects in the body. Instead, phytoestrogens are known for binding to estrogen receptor sites, preventing excess estrogen and stimulating the production of progesterone, thus balancing the hormonal ratios and even serving as anti-estrogens in some cases.

When to use it: Extracts of red clover are well suited for those experiencing menopausal symptoms, especially hot flashes. The rich mineral content is ideal for treatment and prevention of osteoporosis.

The herb is also used topically for rashes and eczema like skin concerns. When made into a cream, it is an excellent substitute for hydrocortisone creams.

Culinary Medicine: Red clover is typically taken as an herbal tea, but not in other dietary preparations.

Optimal Dose: Red clover tea is made with 1 teaspoon of dried herb and flower to an eight ounce glass of water up to three times a day.

When to avoid it: Phytoestrogens may interact both positively and negatively with hormone replacement therapy, so it is best to consult with a professional before combining the two remedies. The herb also has milk blood thinning properties so those taking or avoiding blood thinners should consult with a professional prior to use. Pregnant and breastfeeding should also avoid the herb.

Rosemary
(Rosmarinus officinalis)

Rosemary is a bushy, evergreen shrub native to the Mediterranean, perhaps best known as the herb of remembrance. The most effective and common uses of the herb are to enhance brain function and boost memory abilities. As a result, headaches, tension and stress are all reduced. These benefits are well documented both scientifically and historically, as the ancient Greeks were said to wear garlands of rosemary around their necks during examination to enhance memory and cognitive function.

When to use it: Rosemary is ideal for any individual that could benefit from enhanced brain functioning, whether it be an elderly grandparent suffering from dementia or a college student hitting the books for exam week.

The herb is well suited for both culinary preparations and as an essential extract for diffusion throughout a room. A homeschool or schoolroom setting could benefit greatly from a room diffuser with rosemary oil. The herb also offers valuable antidepressant benefits, so diffusion throughout an office would be a great, inexpensive way to boost productivity and reduce the number of sick days.

Topical application of the extract or oil is also beneficial at stimulating the growth of new hair during hair loss or thinning. It can be added easily to the existing shampoo routine.

Culinary Medicine: Rosemary is a versatile herb, benefiting just about any dish. It is great as an addition to savory brunch dishes, but also adds a boost to any vegetable or meat entrée. When the dish is baked or cooked for a long time, the scent can be released throughout the room offering benefits not unlike that of oil diffusion.

Rosemary Roasted Potatoes
1/4 cup rosemary
1/4 cup olive oil
1/2 teaspoon sea salt and white pepper
3-4 cups halved or quartered new potatoes
Toss the potatoes with the oil and spices. Place into a shallow dish and bake at 400 degrees for 45-50 minutes or until potatoes are tender and beginning to brown around the edges.

Optimal Dose: For a standard 1:5 tincture, up to 10 ml can be taken up to three times a day. However, rosemary is well suited as a culinary herb, so in lieu of dosing by extract, the herb can simply be added liberally to the diet to boost memory and concentration.

When to avoid it: Rosemary is generally considered to be safe, and there are no known situations that would require avoidance of the herb, although some experts suggest limiting use during pregnancy to culinary preparations.

Sage
(*Salvia officinalis*)

Sage is native to the Mediterranean region and the name is derived from a Latin word meaning "to be saved". As expected, it was considered a virtual cure-all, benefiting nearly every disorder.

Currently, research shows that sage is beneficial for treating menopausal complaints, including hot flashes and night sweats. It is also beneficial as a digestive aid and for treating viral and fungal infections.

One surprising use of the herb is as a sweat inhibiting agent. This makes it very popular in natural deodorants and foot creams.

When to use it: Sage is well suited as a supplement for menopausal symptoms. As a culinary herb, it can be added liberally to the diet, and taken as a supplement during times of increased need.

The extract and oil make a good addition to homemade cosmetics, especially those designed for the feet or underarms. In other household uses, sage offers potent cleaning properties, making it suitable as an addition for household cleaners.

Culinary Medicine: Sage is a great example of a medicinal culinary herb. When added to our food, it promotes fresh breath, treating halitosis, and helps to regulate intestinal flora. The herb is very versatile, and can offer tasty benefits to just about any dish at any time of the day.

Baked Eggs with Ricotta and Sage
8 eggs
1 cup ricotta cheese
2 tablespoons sage
1 tablespoon parsley
3 tablespoons Panko breadcrumbs
In a glass measuring cup, whisk the eggs together with the cheese and spices. Divide among 8 small ramekins. Top with the Panko breadcrumbs and bake in a 400 degree oven for 8-10 minutes, or until the eggs are set.

Optimal Dose: As a culinary herb, sage can be added liberally to the diet regularly for optimal benefits. For a tea preparation 2-3 g of the herb is ideal for an eight ounce glass of water. Medicinal amounts of the herb are not recommended for extended use.

When to avoid it: Pregnant and breastfeeding women should limit their use of the herb to culinary purposes.

Saw palmetto
(*Serenoa repens*)

Saw palmetto is a low growing palm tree native to North America, especially Florida. The berries of the tree have a long history for use with male troubles, particularly prostate inflammation, erectile dysfunction and testicular atrophy. It also treats urinary problems in men and hormonal imbalances in women with PCOS.

When to use it: Saw palmetto is a reliable treatment for men with BPH or most other prostate or urinary problems. The herb helps to regulate the production of androgen and brings relief in as little as a month for many men, although complete relief can take longer.

Women with PCOS (polycystic ovarian syndrome) may also benefit form the use of the herb, as it regulates androgen production, which is a cause of many related problems.

Culinary Medicine: Saw palmetto is not often used in culinary preparations, although Dr. James Duke recommends making a pumpkin seed butter with extracts of saw palmetto as a dietary treatment for prostate problems.

Optimal Dose: In a 1:2 extract, 25-30 drops per day can be divided into 2-3 doses.

When to avoid it: Saw palmetto is generally considered to be safe, and there are no known situations that would require avoidance of the herb.

Slippery elm bark
(Ulmus fulva)

Slippery elm bark is native to North America and has been used throughout history as a nutrient and demulcent. George Washing and his troops consumed the bark to provide themselves nutrients during the harsh winter at Valley Forge, and it remains a winter herb to this day, thanks to its soothing actions on the throat that has been irritated by a cough or respiratory infection.

When to use it: Slippery elm bark contains a substance called mucilage, which coats the throat, relieving irritation and helping to reduce coughing spells. To work effectively, it needs to be directly applied to the throat, so encapsulated preparations or extracts will not be effective. The best way to take slippery elm bark is through a tablet that dissolves in the mouth.

Culinary Medicine: Slippery elm bark offers a similar nutritional profile to that of oatmeal, although the intake of gruel seems to have diminished greatly in our modern society. It does, however offer many benefits to the malnourished individual, although finding a suitable preparation may prove to be difficult.

Optimal Dose: Two to three teaspoons of the dried powder are sufficient for one day; this would be equivalent to 1-2 tablets every 3-5 waking hours.

When to avoid it: Slippery elm bark is generally considered to be safe, and there are no known situations that would require avoidance of the herb.

Thyme
(*Thymus vulgaris*)

Thyme holds a place in the history of many ancient cultures. In Egypt, it was used as an embalming agent. The Greeks used its aroma to fill their temples and young women of medieval times gave thyme scented scarves to their knights as a sign of their bravery.

This romantic use did not stop the herb from earning a prominent place in medicine, however. Thyme is a very popular medicinal herb, suitable for culinary use and effective at treating many ailments.

Internally, the herb offers antibacterial properties, helping to regulate the intestinal flora, benefiting gastric complaints. It also has the ability to protect and even increase the amount of DHA in the brain and heart, which then affects many systems and disorders in a positive manner.

It also offers great benefits for respiratory infections, most notably whooping cough and RSV.

When to use it: Thyme can be liberally added to the diet during times of respiratory infection for a reduction in the severity in coughing spells and to help the body "cough up" the trapped mucus.

It is also a great addition to the diet for any child facing ADHD or pregnant women with a developing baby in the womb.

Culinary Medicine: Thyme is well suited for culinary medicine, as it blends well with any of our other Mediterranean herbs.

Savory Thyme Biscuits
2 cups flour
1 tablespoon baking soda
1 tablespoon baking powder
1 teaspoon salt
1 stick butter
3/4 cup buttermilk
1 egg
2 tablespoons thyme
2 tablespoons sun dried tomatoes, chopped
1/4 cup shredded cheddar cheese
Combine dry ingredients. Make a well in the center and add wet ingredients. Stir until just combined. (You will need to use your hands for this part.) Scoop by heaping tablespoons onto a greased baking sheet. Bake at 400 degrees for 14 or 15 minutes until lightly browned. Serve with additional butter. For a hearty breakfast, fill with a fried egg or slice of breakfast meat, or both!

Optimal Dose: Tea made with thyme contains 1-2 teaspoons of the dried herb per 8 ounces of water.

When to avoid it: Pregnant women should restrict the use of thyme to culinary purposes only.

Uvi ursi
(*Actosostaphylos uva ursi)*

This evergreen perennial shrub, also known as bearberry, is native to the northern hemisphere, including North America, Europe and Asia. While it did not make its medical debut until quite recently for herbs (circa 1600AD), it has become a staple for treatment of urinary tract and kidney infections over the last few hundred years.

When to use it: Uva ursi is best taken at the onset or diagnosis of an urinary tract infection or kidney infection. It prevents bacteria from adhering to the lining of the urinary tract, and is effective as an antibacterial agent against *E. coli,* a common cause of urinary tract infections.

The medicinal compounds responsible for this action are not readily extracted in water, so extracts are the ideal source of treatment with uva ursi.

Culinary Medicine: Uva ursi is not an herb that is used for culinary purposes.

Optimal Dose: In a 1:1 extract, 3ml of uva ursi can be taken up to four times a day.

When to avoid it: Uva Ursi is not suitable for pregnant women, breastfeeding women, children under the age of 12 years or for prolonged use. It should be taken by non pregnant, non breastfeeding adults for short terms, until the infection has cleared.

Section Four:
The Natural Family Toolkit

Harvesting Medicinal Herbs

Many of our medicinal herbs can easily be grown at home for personal use. Not only is this a productive skill, it is quite fun and rewarding. When harvested and stored correctly, these herbs can provide many benefits in the natural home.

The first step in choosing herbs to harvest is to carefully evaluate the plant. While herb walks and plucking wild plants used to be the ideal solution and the norm, modern use of heavy pesticides and herbicides has made this a difficult task. Unless you are very familiar with the land and its history, I do not recommend searching for medicinal or culinary herbs in the wild.

Next, we need to ensure that the plant is free of rot, pests and overripe fruits. The best health benefits come from healthy plants. Plants that are struggling to survive are not going to be the best source of medicinal properties and healthy nutrients.

When to Harvest

Flowers should be picked on a warn day in the mid morning. Ideally, the dew should have had ample time to dry off, but the heat of the day should not have set in yet. For the best results, the flowers should have recently blossomed. After collecting, they can be placed in a cooling rack or small screen to dry.

Bark should be harvested in the spring or fall. It should be cut into small strips so that it can dry easily and not run a chance of molding.

Seeds should be collected when the plant ripens, after it is fully grown.

Leaves, like flowers, are harvested in the middle of the morning. The dew should already have dried, but the heat has not yet set in. Unlike flowers, however, leaves should be picked before the plant buds or begins to flower. Instead of picking individual leaves, the whole stem is picked and dried, then the leaves are removed after the stem is dry.

Roots should be harvested according to their type. Perennial plants should be harvested in the fall after the plant is dormant, but before the first frost has arrived. If this ideal season has been missed, they can also be harvested in the early spring, after the last frost. Biennials are harvested in the fall of the first year or spring of the second year. The key is to remember to harvest it before it has begun to grow plenty of foliage. Roots are cut into small chunks for drying.

Sometimes the whole herb is harvested. In these cases, they should be picked when the flowers are just beginning to bloom, in the morning after the dew has dried and before the hottest part of the day. These plants are dried whole, then cut and sifted once fully dry.

Drying the Herbs

While many herbs can be used fresh, drying the herb allows it to be stored and saved for use throughout the year. However, if left alone, the water content can cause the plant to mold, become contaminated with bacteria and change the chemical composition of the plant, rendering it useless for culinary and medicinal purposes. For these reasons, the herbs should be properly dried if they will not be put to immediate use. It is also important to note that some herbs, especially many barks, should be aged for a year or longer before using to prevent harsh side effects.

The best way to dry herbs is to place them onto a screen or cooling rack. The rack should be placed in a warm area with plenty of fresh air circulating throughout. It should also be placed out of direct sunlight.

When dry, the herb will weigh less than half of the original weight. While the herb should be fully dry, it should not become brittle or crumbly.

Storing the Herbs

The dried herbs must also be properly stored to preserve the beneficial properties. It is important to remember that air and light speed the oxidation of the herb, so avoidance of these two factors is crucial.

To accomplish this, herbs should be placed in dark glass containers or clear glass stored in a dark cabinet. The containers should be filled completely or filled with cotton or muslin to fill the leftover space. These containers should be stored between 55 and 70 degrees. Hotter or cooler temperatures can affect the chemical reactions in the plant matter.

Once stored, flowers, leaves, whole herbs and fruits can be kept an average of 12 months, then should be discarded and replaced with fresh. Roots, however, can be kept up to 30 months before they have to be replaced.

A New Vocabulary

Adaptogen: An adaptogen is an herb that can boost the body's immune response, and increase resistance to stress, fatigue, trauma, and anxiety.

Allopathic: Allopathic medicine is the popular modern system of medicine. In a broad, general sense, allopathic medicine focuses on treating illness after it happens and relies heavily on treating symptoms with pharmaceuticals.

Botanical Medicine: Botanical medicine is another term for herbal medicine. Botanical or herbal medicine generally rely on the principles of holistic care and feature plant extracts or remedies for helping the body heal itself.

Compress: A compress is a tool for applying herbal remedies topically. Generally, a compress can be made with a warm cloth, moistened with an infusion of the herb.

Constituent, active: The active constituent is the part of the herb that contains the most medicinal value.

Doula: A doula is a non medical birth assistant. The most common type of doula assists the expecting family (particularly the mother and father to be) with preparation for the birth, and helps the mother throughout the labor, delivery and immediate postpartum period. She brings an extensive working knowledge of birth procedures and techniques, natural pain relief measures and advanced comfort measures for the mother. According to research, the doula can dramatically reduce the occurrence of epidural use, induction measures (such as artificial hormones), forceps use and cesarean rates. The doula works in addition to the obstetrician or midwife.

Extract: Extract is a term that can include both tinctures and glycerties. The term does not distinguish between the possible liquids used to extract the medicinal properties of the herb, it simply refers to the extracted substance.

Flexitarian: A flexitarian is an individual that recognizes the importance of a plant based diet, but still chooses to consume meat on limited occasions, such as holidays or other celebrations. The flexitarian lifestyle is a middle ground for those that would like to be vegetarians, but choose to occasionally consume animal products for health reasons, or even simple convenience.

Flora: The term flora describes the living organisms in the digestive tract, namely yeasts and bacteria. They exist in a symbiotic relationship, that is greatly affected by antibiotics, birth control pills and other substances.

Gluten: Gluten is the main protein matrix in wheat and many other grains. While it is an obvious benefit, as a vegetarian protein source, it can cause harm to many that are intolerant or allergic to gluten. Many children with autism or ADHD show benefit when gluten is removed from the diet, and those with Celiac disease must avoid gluten indefinitely.

Glycerite: A glycerite is an herbal extract that contains vegetable glycerin as the main ingredient. Some glycerites actually used glycerin as the extracting agent, while others used alcohol to extract the medicinal properties then went through a process to remove the alcohol, replacing it with glycerin. Glycerites are ideal for children, alcoholics and adults with sensitive stomachs, as the glycerin is a mild, almost sweet substance, while alcohol has a sting or burn to it.

Greenwashing: Greenwashing refers to the popular practice of marketing a product as providing green benefits, when it actually does not. This is usually a simple result of stretching the truth or overstating the potential benefits of a product.

Herbalist: An herbalist is an individual that has extensive training in the values of plants and the basics of natural health. While many herbalists are self trained, it is often ideal to choose an herbalist that has completed a thorough herbal training program or experienced an apprenticeship with an advanced herbalist. Herbalists do not practice medicine, rather they consult with clients and work in a partnership with the physician or care provider.

Holistic: Holistic is the term used to describe the type of care that views the body or individual as a whole, not merely a group of unrelated parts. Many prefer to use the term wholistic.

Homeopathy: Homeopathy is a form of natural medicine based on three principles: like cures like, minimal dose and single remedy. While the two systems often use the same source, it is not the same as herbalism or botanical medicine.

Midwife: A midwife is an individual trained and experienced in providing care to women during the childbearing years. Certified midwives have demonstrated competency in both low risk birth and unexpected complications. Depending on the type of midwife and the state, midwives deliver babies in both hospital and home settings, as well as natural birth centers, which form a bridge between the two.

Natural: This term is becoming more and more popular in marketing and advertising, but is unregulated, and can literally mean anything. It is a prime example of greenwashing, as our grocers are filled with naturally fitting diapers, cleaners and body care with natural ingredients (in addition to the many harmful ones, however) and natural food items, that contain dozens of artificially produced additives.

Organic: Organic is a term used to describe foods that have been grown without the use of pesticides, artificial fertilizers and genetic modification. The term is regulated, so the term is somewhat more reliable than "natural".

Probiotic: A probiotic is a strand of beneficial bacteria that helps to protect the intestine from harmful bacteria. Probiotics are found in fermented foods and can be taken as a supplement.

Supplement: A supplement is a substance taken in addition to the diet that offers health benefits to the individual. Vitamins, minerals and herbs are all regulated as health supplements.

Tincture: A tincture is an extract that contains the herbal constituents in an alcohol base. It is a concentrated solution,

A Few of My Favorite Things

There are many wonderful sources for products that a natural family can use. This list is by means exhaustive, but the sources listed here are personal favorites in the Hawkins' home.

Vintage Remedies Website / Ebooks
The Vintage Remedies website (www.VintageRemedies.com) contains a wealth of information from gluten free and whole foods recipes to tips on living a natural life well. The site is updated weekly with more great tips and formulas.

American Herbalists Guild / Journal
The Journal of the American Herbalist Guild contains a wealth of herbal information for the aspiring professional. It is a benefit of membership, which is a must for any herbalist-to-be.

Atlantic Spice
This is a good source of bulk herbs, a few essential oils and some useful natural tools such as tea bags and muslin bags. While the selection may not be as vast as some other sources, the quality is reliable, and the service is impeccable. www.AtlanticSpice.com

Flora Health

Many of my favorite herbal products are manufactured by Flora Health, including the iron supplements Floradix and Floravital and FlorEssence, a gentle detoxification formula. Additionally, their website contains monographs on many of the herbs they use in their formulas and detailed information on their products. www.FloraHealth.com

Frontier Co-op

The wholesale Frontier co-op is a wonderful resource for purchasing large amounts of natural living essentials. We have received fantastic service and a vast selection of products that are essential for the healthy home. www.FrontierCoop.com

Herbalgram / American Botanical Council

The American Botanical Council is a non profit research organization that offers reliable information about herbs and the latest scientific research. Their membership website provides a complete version of the Commission E monographs (translated into English) and their quarterly journal, *Herbalgram,* provides useful information for the professional or aspiring herbalist. www.Herbalgram.org

Herbs for Health

This is the perfect herbal magazine for the newcomer or the herbalist that enjoys reading fun and practical material. www.HerbsforHealth.com

Mountain Rose Herbs

While I cannot vouch for the line of reading material they offer, Mountain Rose Herbs carries an extensive line of dried herbs and essential oils. I purchase most of my herbs in bulk from them and have always received wonderful service. www.MountainRoseHerbs.com

Something Better Natural Foods

This is another coop we frequently use. They offer dried food products, and are a reliable source of grains, rice and other healthy foods, with an abundance of organic varieties. www.SomethingBetterNaturalFoods.com

Vitacost.com

Vitacost is a great resource for name brand remedies at discounted prices. They carry nearly every one of my favorite brands and have fast and reasonable shipping.

Natural Cleaning

Air fresheners

Air fresheners are a common cause of toxin accumulation in the home. Some natural health experts have even gone as far as to compare the damage of conventional air fresheners with that of cigarette smoke! These natural fresheners are a much safer option with therapeutic benefits.

1/2 cup vodka
1/2 cup distilled water
15 drops essential oils (see below)

> **calming:** 8 drops lavender / 4 drops geranium / 3 drops lemon
> **deodorizing:** 8 drops lavender / 4 drops clove / 3 drops lemon
> **minty:** 8 drops peppermint / 6 drops spearmint / 1 drop orange
> **holiday spice:** 5 drops cinnamon / 5 drops clove / 5 drops orange
> **springtime**: 6 drops lavender / 5 drops orange / 4 drops rose

Combine all ingredients together with the oil blend of your choice in a spray bottle. Cap and shake well.

Antibacterial Spray

When illness is lingering from person to person in the same household, it is time for some serious antibacterial cleansing. This spray is ideal for toilet handles, light switches, doorknobs, phones, and anything else that is frequently touched be everyone in the home.

1/2 cup distilled water
1/2 cup vodka
25 drops orange oil
15 drops lavender oil
15 drops eucalyptus oil

Mix well and store in a spray bottle. Shake prior to use.

Basic Laundry Soap

Not only does this laundry soap smell great, it is all natural and gentle enough even for baby clothes. The Vintage Remedies cleaning kits and workshops use the lavender lemon blend of essential oil for this formula, which helps to remove stains, freshen and brighten the laundry and adds a subtle fresh scent to the load.

Mix together 6-8 T vegetable soap, 3.5 cups of baking soda, either the borax or washing soda (see below) and 2 cups of warm distilled water. Add 35 drops essential oil blend. Use 2-4 T per load
For hard water, add 1/2 cup –3/4 cups of borax. For normal water, add 1/2 –3/4 cups of washing soda or additional baking soda.

Citrus Soft Scrubbing Paste

This thick paste is perfect for scrubbing tubs, showers, tile and other flat surfaces. The citrus oils help to cut grease and kill germs. Like all scouring pastes, always check a small area first, to ensure the surface is up to the scrubbing!

1 cup baking soda
1/4 cup vegetable soap

1 T distilled water
20 drops essential oil blend (equal parts orange, lemon, lime)

Mix thoroughly. Add 1 T distilled vinegar (it might foam a bit) and stir until smooth. Scoop into an airtight jar, cap and label. (Note: after long storage, the mixture may become dry. This can be remedied by adding distilled water 1 T at a time.)

Fabric Softener

1 cup vinegar
15 drops lavender oil
25 drops lemon oil

Combine thoroughly and pour 2T into the fabric softener compartment of the washing machine, or use a time release ball.

Foaming Carpet Cleaner

When all of these ingredients are tossed into the blender, a thick foam forms, which is perfect for cleaning carpets yet gentle enough for the whole family, even children to play on.

Simply take 2 cups of water and add 1/2 cup of vegetable soap. Toss in 10-12 drops of your favorite essential oil (a strong one like peppermint works well) Blend until foamy. Remove and scoop onto the carpet, rubbing in a circular motion. Wipe with a damp cloth.

Four Thieves Anti-Plague Formula

While the legend changes as much as the formula for this historic blend, the gist of the story is this: During the plagues (enter your favorite plague here, the Black Plague is most common, but the tale has even made its way to America, as a plague that struck New Orleans), a family began robbing the dead. At first, they were largely ignored, as everyone knew they would eventually pay the price by catching the plague themselves, but they managed to avoid it. When finally captured, the judge wanted to know how they avoided the plague, but they refused. After much debating, they agreed to share their secret in return for their pardon. The secret was that they were the offspring of a perfumer and herbalist. They knew these oils would protect them so they rubbed them on their bodies and used them to clean anything they brought back. The powerful blend is also often called the Grave Robbers Blend

1 cup vinegar
15 drops rosemary oil
15 drops lavender oil
15 drops sage oil
15 drops peppermint oil
20 drops lemon oil
10 drops eucalyptus oil

The formula can be changed, and has been altered often. The key ingredients are mint, lavender, rosemary and sage. These have been assisted by many an herbalist that feels he or she can improve upon the basic formula. Garlic is often added, and many others like to add tinctures to make a formula that is taken internally. Due to the potent nature of the mix, I do not recommend taking internally. I prefer to stick to original use, according to the legends, which is that of a cleaning product.

Freshening Powder

This quick and easy recipe can be used to freshen sheets, carpets, or even couches. Simply sprinkle on, then vacuum off. It may take more than one trip with the vacuum to catch it all, but each time will release more of the oils into the air. (We obviously don't vacuum our sheets! If the powder is used for sheets or delicate upholstery, a light sprinkling sans vacuuming will do.)

Simply take 1 cup of baking soda and add 10-12 drops of essential oil of choice. Store in an airtight container between uses.

Gentle Baby Laundry Soap

Most natural soaps are gentle enough for a baby's delicate skin. Yet, there is just something about having a specially formulated soap just for baby, complete with soothing and gentle essential oil fragrance. This formula is one of the most gentle formulas for washing laundry, yet is still potent enough to get out those organic baby stains.

1/2 cup washing soda
2 cups baking soda
1/2 cup vegetable soap (liquid)
15 drops lavender oil (optional)
1 cup distilled water

Blend all ingredients together thoroughly. Use 3-4T per average size load.

Minty Window Wash

Even if you despise cleaning windows, we can all agree that there is nothing like the pristine view of nature just outside that is not inhibited by streaks or little handprints! Like the rest of my home, I clean my windows with natural cleaners that won't emit harmful fumes into the air that my children breathe. My favorite window formula is this minty one, which offers a perky mint fragrance. Mint also helps to deter pests, which makes it ideal for a window or glass door that may otherwise be attractive to pests looking for an entrance.

In a spray bottle, combine:
5 drops spearmint oil
4 drops peppermint oil
1/2 cup distilled vinegar
2T vodka
1/2 cup distilled water

Shake well to ensure all contents are thoroughly distributed. Spray onto the window and wash or wipe as usual.

Quick Disinfecting Spray

Sometimes we simply don't have the time to whip up a batch of homemade cleaners, but we need the house clean nonetheless. This cleaner can be thrown together in literally seconds, leaving plenty of time for cleaning.

1 cup vinegar
15 drops lavender oil

Combine the two in a spray bottle and use anywhere you would normally use a disinfectant.

Tough Stain Remover

This is an excellent choice for both laundry and upholstery stains. It is simple to make in a hurry, and uses everyday household ingredients. What else can we ask for?

Take 1-2 T cream of tarter and mix in 3-4 drops peppermint essential oil. Thin with 1-3 t of water until it reaches your desired texture. Rub into the stain or store in an airtight container.

Tub and Tile Cleaning Paste

This is ideal for any solid surface and helps break down soap scum and other common troubles. If it begins to dry out, simply add a few drops of water and stir well.

1 cup baking soda
1/4 cup vegetable soap
1 T distilled water
1 T vinegar
20 drops essential oil blend of choice (Citrus oils make a great choice for this as they are effective de-greasers.)

Mix together the soda and soap. Add the water and essential oils. When thoroughly combined, stir in the vinegar. The mixture may foam a little. Scoop into a clean jar, cap and label.

Wooden Floor Polish

Most floors no longer need polishing, but in case you are fortunate to come across a solid wood floor that does require it, this wax is tough to beat.

1/4 cup olive oil
1 ounce beeswax
12 drops lavender oil

Melt the wax into the oil until just mixed. As the mixture begins to cool, stir in the lavender and continue stirring vigorously until a creamy semi solid mass appears. Scoop into a tin for storage.

Indulging Skin Care

Chocolate Chip Bath Cookies

During one of my pregnancies, I taught classes at the local recreation center on how to make natural body care products. One of the biggest hits was the tween class when we made these bath cookies. Every one of them listed this single project as their favorite. Since then, I have made these cookies with girls at princess birthday parties, as a scouting project, and even as a youth Sunday School "girls night out" craft. the uses are limitless and girls of all ages love tossing these fizzy chocolate scented treats into the bath!

You will need: a pinch of copper and black mica powder, a pinch of cocoa powder, 1/2 cup of baking soda, 1/4 cup of citric acid, 1/2 cup milk powder or ground oats (oats will give your dough a more natural look), 1 ounce cocoa butter, melted, 1/4 cup glycerin, and 1/4 cup large bath salts. (The baking soda, milk powder, ground oats and citric acid can be found at the local grocer. Cocoa butter and glycerin can be found at a health food store, and the salts and mica powders will have to be purchased through an online supplier that stocks body care product ingredients.)

Mix salts, mica powders and cocoa together with a few drops of glycerin until well blended. Set aside.

Mix all remaining dry ingredients, then slowly add the wet ingredients. Fold in the "chocolate chips" and scoop into small balls. Let dry overnight.

Clean and Green Mask

This mask is ideal for offering soothing benefits as well as deep pore cleansing. Avocados oxidize quickly, so make the mask right before using and do not store the leftovers. The clay helps to draw toxins out of the skin and avocados soothe and gently exfoliate the tender area.

1/4 cup white clay
1 avocado

Peel and seed the avocado. Save half for another use. In a small bowl, mash the avocado and the powder together until a paste forms. If necessary, add 1-2 t distilled water until desired consistency is reached. Massage into the face and neck area and allow to sit for 3-5 minutes. Rinse off with a warm cloth and moisturize, if needed.

Cleopatra's Bath

Rumor has it that Cleopatra had the most beautiful skin. After studying her historic accomplishments, she certainly had to have something going for her! Using her ancient bathing secrets, if nothing else, we will have soft and moisturized skin. This bath calls for some difficult ingredients, but the final product is worthy of the trouble.

1 cup milk powder (organic is best)
1/2 cup cocoa butter shavings
1/4 cup oatmeal powder (to powder oats, give them a whir in the blender for about 20 seconds)
2/3 cup Epsom salts
25 drops ylang ylang oil
35 drops sweet orange oil

Combine the salts and oils in a small bowl. In a larger bowl, mix together the remaining ingredients. Add the salt / oil blend and stir well to combine. Place in a decorative jar. To use, scoop out 1/3 cup into a warm bath. The water will melt the cocoa butter creating a fragrant, soothing and moisturizing bath.

Coconut Vanilla Body Butter

This moisture laden crème is so soothing after a long day on the beach or in the hot sun. Make sure the coconut oil is virgin or the scent will not be strong enough.

1/2 cup virgin coconut oil
15 drops pure vanilla glycerine extract
1/4 cup grapeseed oil
1 T beeswax

Stir together all of the ingredients omitting the vanilla. Warm over gentle heat until the beeswax is melted. Remove and stir every 3-4 minutes as it cools to prevent separation. When the mixture begins to thicken, add the vanilla and blend well. Store in a cool place during warm weather to prevent rancidity and keep a creamy texture. Use within 2-3 months.

Esther's Ancient Beauty Secret

As we see through the Biblical account of Esther, ancient beauty routines were intricate and elaborate. Very few of the actual formulas and details have survived over time, but this formula is said to date back to the ancient harems of old. We know that the beautification process like what Esther went through involved luxurious baths, henna art and a skin enhancing paste much like this one. (Note: this recipe makes enough for two applications)

1 T orange peel, dried and ground
3 T ground almonds
2 T oats
1/8 t of ground cloves

1 T ground dried rose petals
1/8 t nutmeg (ground)
2 T sweet almond oil
6 drops neroli
6 drops sandalwood

Mix all ingredients together until a paste forms. Add a drop or two of additional almond oil, if needed. Unlike the other scrubs, this one is applied to freshly cleansed skin. After bathing, dry off and roll the paste all over the body. Massage it into the skin, leaving a sheer coating of the paste. After the entire amount has been massaged in, begin to wipe off any dried excess from the skin.

Footsies Scrub

The Footsies line of foot care was one of Swaddle Spa's most popular products. While the original formula makes a huge batch and requires some difficult to obtain ingredients, this version has been adapted to be produced easily in the kitchen. This scrub is for the feet any time of the year, but especially in the summer when they are often exposed to the elements in our skimpy sandals and "flip flops". The peppermint oil is invigorating and stimulating, and the exfoliating properties keep them smooth and fresh.

1 cup sea salts, finely ground
1/4 cup grapeseed oil
10-12 drops peppermint essential oil

Stir together the oils. Pour in the salt, 1/4 cup at a time, blending well after each addition. For a softer scent, substitute 5-6 drops spearmint oil for half of the peppermint. Scoop into a sterile dish and seal. To use, scoop out 2-3 T and scrub the feet and lower calves well. Rinse off, taking care not to slip, as the oils coat and moisturize the feet. Use within 2-3 months.

Honey and Oats Mask

Oatmeal and honey is a classic combination across farms everywhere. These fresh ingredients make a warming breakfast cereal, but perform even better in the home spa cabinet. The mask is simple to make and has many beneficial properties. The oats soothe irritated skin. As they are massaged into the delicate facial area, they gentle exfoliate, removing dead skin cells, and and anti-inflammatory properties are increasingly valuable.

When we add honey to the mix we get a natural humectant, which means it helps to draw moisture to the skin, leaving it nice and hydrated. The natural scents of the ingredients combine to leave a caramel like fragrance in the air, but they can be deepened by the addition of a drop or two of vanilla extract. This mask is best made right before applying to the skin, so double or triple the formula for a crowd.

2 T honey
1/4 cup oats

Grind the oats in a blender until they are coarsely chopped, but not powdered. Place in a small bowl and drizzle the honey over the top. Add the vanilla if using. With your hands, combine until a rough paste forms and spread across the skin. Leave on the face for 4-5 minutes and rinse with warm water. Be sure to remove all of the honey. Finish with a moisturizer.

Lavender Lemon Bath Salts

These salts contain Epsom salts to soothe tired muscles after an active day of fun. The relaxing scent offers just the right amount of soothing yet stimulating properties to help you recover. The herbs also make a pretty presentation. Make sure to put these in a clear jar to show off the light colors.

1 cup epsom salts
1 cup coarse sea salts
2 T dried lavender buds

2 T lemon zest
12 drops lemon essential oil
7 drops lavender essential oil
Blend all ingredients together, making sure the oils are well incorporated. Scoop into an airtight jar and scoop 1/4 to 1/2 cup of salts into a warm bath. (Optional: Scoop salts into a muslin tea bag to keep the herbs contained.)

Lavender Petals Sugar Scrub

Powdery white sugar is not what I consider a healthy food, but it is a useful ingredient to have in my home spa kit. I put it to good use in this white and purple speckled scrub. With the lavender buds, this makes a pretty decorative gift. The shelf life is shorter than other scrubs, so keep an eye on it. I like to package it in smaller jars, so it is more likely to be used up before it goes bad.

1 cup white sugar
3 T cup refined coconut oil
3 T sweet almond oil
2 T lavender buds
20 drops lavender essential oil

In a small bowl, combine the oils. Scoop onto the mound of sugar and stir until well combined. Stir in the flower buds and package in a shallow jar. To use, massage a small amount into the skin. Rinse. The flower buds will clog a drain, so use sparingly!

Lip Gloss

Every girl, regardless of age loves the fresh feeling of lip gloss, which makes this project fun to make for keeping or giving. The batch easily doubles or triples for holiday giving (or stocking up on flavors!) The slippery castor oil is responsible for the glossy effect.

1 t beeswax
1 T cocoa butter
1 T coconut oil

1 t castor oil

Combine in a small glass jar and place in the oven or microwave until melted. Stir in 6-8 drops of sweet orange essential oil and pour into sterile jars or tins. Allow to firm then place a detailed label on the package.

Minty Mornings Shower Gel

I usually consider myself a morning person, but in the dreary wintertime, I often need quite a bit of coaxing to get out to bed and get my day going. My mornings are much easier when I have this body wash on hand in the shower. The energizing scents are uplifting and kick start my day.

1 cup liquid organic castile soap
1/4 cup vegetable glycerin
1/3 cup sweet almond oil
15 drops peppermint oil
10 drops spearmint oil
5 drops sweet orange oil

In a glass mixing bowl, pour all the ingredients. Stir gently to combine. Too much stirring will cause it to bubble over. The mixture will turn cream colored as it combines. Pour into a bottle and enjoy.

Simple Sugar Facial

One of my favorite skin care routines is one of the simplest in the book. This is my back up plan. Whenever my face begins to loose its youthful glow, or become dry (or oily), I rely on this classic formula. The ingredients are always in the house, and even on a busy night, I can toss this together and feel fresh and clean.

Simply take 2-3 T of sugar and place it in your palm. Drizzle about 1-2t olive oil in the center and with the other hand, rub together to make a paste. Using both hands, work the paste over the face, paying special attention to any "problem" areas such as the forehead or chin. Wet a washcloth with hot water. Hold the cloth about 2 inches from your face (be careful not to burn yourself!) As it cools, wipe off the remaining sugar and oil. You may need to rinse a few times to remove any unabsorbed oil. This is best done at night, when you can leave your face free from make up for several hours.

Skin Soothing Soak

Sunburns, rashes, itchy clothing.. it does not take much to make our delicate skin irritated. Fortunately, this soothing soak is just the key to restoring our smooth and clear skin. Make up a batch to keep on hand for when the moment strikes! I like to keep this bright soak in a glass canning jar with a brown cord tied around the top. The bright yellow flowers and white salts make a beautiful rustic, yet clean looking product.

1 cup calendula petals
1 cup chamomile petals
1 cup Epsom salts
5 drops lavender oil

Stir together the essential oil and salt. When it is thoroughly combined (make sure not to leave any clumps of oil), stir in the herbs. Store in a tightly sealed jar. To use: scoop out 1/2 cup and place in a muslin cloth. A tea bag works well, but a cloth can be tied together at the top to prevent the flowers from escaping! Toss into a warm bath and swirl through the water to evenly disperse the infusion.

"Unwind" Bath Salts

Epsom salts are used in this formula for their muscle relaxing properties. Not only do they help the body relax, they are soothing for irritated skin. Regular sea salt is added as well for additional minerals and soothing effects. The essential oil blend deepens this effect, with soothing, relaxing oils. This is the perfect product for a soothing bath after a long hard day.

1 cup Epsom salts
1 cup sea salts

1 T coconut oil
7 drops lavender oil
5 drops

Vanilla Brown Sugar Scrub

Body scrubs have the ability to polish the skin and leave it feeling fresh and smooth. I love the feel of a good sea salt scrub, but the salt can irritate sensitive skin, especially after shaving or when there is a cut or scrape. The use of brown sugar helps to eliminate that potential problem and gives a gentle polish, not a rough scrub. The cocoa butter soothes the skin after scrubbing, leaving it nice and supple. For a vanilla scented scrub, use unscented cocoa butter. For a chocolate scented scrub, use raw cocoa butter.

1.5 cups brown sugar
1/3 cup sweet almond oil
1/4 cup grated cocoa butter
1 t vanilla extract

Pour the sugar into a medium bowl. Drizzle the oil and vanilla over the top, stirring until combined. It will form a thick mass. Stir in the cocoa butter shavings and scoop into a pretty glass jar. This is a good scrub for clear jars, because the color is so appealing.

For Further Learning

Putting natural medicine to use in the home is just like any other part of parenting; it is a learning process. Even professional herbalists and care providers are constantly researching and learning about the latest research, safety considerations and additional remedies that will benefit their family members, clients or patients. This book is certainly not intended to be an "end all" reference for healthy living. To further your knowledge of safe and healthy herbal use in the home, our School of Natural Health is highly recommended.

The Vintage Remedies School of Natural Health offers both Family Herbalist and Master Herbalist programs with distance learning options from a Christian perspective. It is the only program available to do so. Both curriculums were written and compiled by yours truly, and can be purchased through the Vintage Remedies website or by emailing or calling us at the office for more details.

Family Herbalist Program

Research shows that 80% of people turn to a motherly female figure for medical advice prior to calling a medical professional. What do we have to offer them in terms of solid advice? Do we turn to the latest health trend, recite what we saw on TV last night, or do we really have solid, evidence based information to offer? The Vintage Remedies School of Natural Health Family Herbalist program, is designed to train the Family Herbalist in Western herbalism from a Christian perspective. This course will train the family herbalist in areas of prevention, nutrition, body chemistry, anatomy, herbal preparations, aromatherapy, and so much more.

The program contains 26 units, each consisting of a lesson, required reading assignments, a related project and a test, which is submitted for review. There is an additional mid-term test after unit 13 and a final exam after the last unit. Upon completion, a certificate will be issued from the Vintage Remedies School of Natural Health to the graduate as a "Family Herbalist".

The program also includes:

* personal "one on one" time with Jessie Hawkins for study guidance
* access to the "students only" email group
* supply kit with herbs, essential oils and other project supplies

Study Topics include:

Anatomy and Physiology
Wholistic Nutrition
Modern Childhood Epidemics
Creating a Home Medicine Chest
Common Childhood and Adult Illnesses
Herbal Classifications and Pharmacognosy
Herbal Preparations
Materia Medica (130 herbs and oils!)
Aromatherapy
Creating a Wholistic Living Network
and more!

Family Herbalist Course Outline:

1. The Germ vs Terrain Theory
2. Wholistic Nutrition
3. Wholistic Nutrition part 2
4. Bread: The Staff of Life
5. Body Chemistry
6. Healthy Pregnancy and Birthing
7. Prevention the First Year and Beyond
8. Vaccinations
9. Modern Day Childhood Epidemics
10. Pharmacognosy and Herbal Medications
11. Body Systems
12. Herbal Home Use
13. Herbal Preparations part 1
14. Childhood Illness
15. Adult Illness
16. Dealing with Acute or Serious Illness
17. Herbal Classifications
18. Herbal Materia Medica
19. Herbal Materia Medica part 2
20. Herbal Materia Medica part 3
21. Advanced Herbal Preparations
22. Aromatherapy
23. Aromatherapy in the Home
24. Diffusion Methods and Special Needs
25. Prevention in Homekeeping
26. Contacting Outside Help

Master Herbalist Program

The natural health industry is one of the fastest growing industries in the world, with supplement sales reaching billions of dollars in the United States alone. Worldwide, nearly 3/4 of the population rely on "complementary" medicine, while only roughly 1/4 use "conventional" medicine. For example, in Germany, it is estimated that 1 in 3 drugs prescribed is an herb. Furthermore, studies show us that nearly 75% of Americans desire more natural treatments, and repeated published trials conclude that care providers need to become more educated in the area of complimentary medicine.

Unfortunately, there is an abundance of misinformation available on the topic, and studies also show us that roughly 2/3 of the individuals currently taking herbal supplements are not using them correctly. There is an urgent need for well educated experts in this emerging new field, and this need is growing daily.

This is exactly why the Master Herbalist program at the Vintage Remedies School of Natural Health was created. This mastery program covers all aspects of natural health, from defining the scope of your profession to setting up and marketing your new business. With the Family Herbalist certificate as a prerequisite, the entire program offers a complete education including nutrition, aromatherapy, pharmacognosy, anatomy, elements of wellness, body chemistry, modern disease, plant identification and harvesting, the mind body connection, legal considerations and much, much more.

Graduates will leave the program with a certificate as a Master Herbalist and are granted permission to use the Vintage Remedies materials, handouts and affiliation.

The Master Herbalist program is available in the same user friendly format that we offer for our Family Herbalist program. There are 40 units, each self paced and suitable for incremental learning.

Like the Family Herbalist Course, the Master Herbalist program also includes:

Personal one on one time with Jessie for feedback and input
Access to the students only online group
Ongoing assistance and guidance as a professional herbalist

1. History and Philosophy of Herbal Medicine
2. Evidenced Based Medicine
3. Concepts of Advanced Phytotherapy
4. Botany / Plant Anatomy
5. Herbal Identification
6. Plants as Whole Food
7. Medical Terminology
8. Phytopharmaceutical Terminology
9. Adaptogens
10. General Pharmacology
11. Toxicity and Contraindications
12. Reactions and Interactions
13. Advanced Aromatherapy
14. Circulatory System
15. Digestive System
16. Endocrine System
17. Materia Medica I
18. Lymphatic System
19. Integumentary System
20. Muscular System
21. Materia Medica II
22. Nervous System
23. Respiratory System
24. Urinary System
25. Materia Medica III
26. Female Reproductive System
27. Male Reproductive System
28. Materia Medica IV
29. Phytotherapy for Gestation and Lactation
30. Pediatric Phytotherapy
31. Geriatric Phytotherapy
32. Advanced Wholistic Nutrition
33. Client Intake Strategies
34. Nutritional Consulting
35. Wellness Consulting
36. Lectures, Seminars and Workshops
37. Legal Jurisprudence
38. Career Development / Ethics / Record Keeping
39. Marketing for the Herbal Consultant
40. Final

Appendix One: A Word About Antibiotic Overuse taken from the July 2007 Vintage Remedies newsletter

Antibiotics, the wonder drug of the 1940's, are thought by many to be a virtual miracle worker for any and every ailment. When surveyed, most people believe that antibiotics are beneficial for both bacterial and viral infections, and that they can even benefit colds and the flu. Many moms still believe antibiotics are not only beneficial but necessary during an ear infection and that they are harmless for their children. Studies show that roughly 40% of the time children leave the physician's office, moms leave with a prescription for an antibiotic.

Unfortunately, antibiotics are not the harmless wonder workers capable of curing every problem that comes our (or our child's) way. The overuse of this potent drug is not only a matter of living naturally or trying herbal medications, but an important issue of safety and potential danger. Antibiotics can only help with bacterial infections. Not only do they offer nothing for viral infections, many studies show they actually lead to longer healing times and recurring cases. Even when used for bacterial infections, they can often be overused, which leads to antibiotic resistant bacteria.

Antibiotic resistant bacteria is nothing new. The issue first arose within a few years of mainstream use, after antibiotics were added to cough drops and even lotions. Finally regulated to prescription use, the need still existed and continues to exist for stronger antibiotics. Antibiotic resistance is, according to the CDC, one of the most pressing problems the world faces face today. So pressing that the CDC has launched a national campaign, known as the "Get Smart" Campaign, promoting more appropriate use of antibiotics by physicians and parents. According to the CDC, tens of millions of antibiotics are prescribed in physician's offices annually for viral infections. One of the main reason cited by the physicians as the reason for prescribing the antibiotics was patient demand. (Date: August 29, 2006
Content source: National Center for Immunization and Respiratory Diseases/Division of Bacterial Diseases)

What can we do as parents and patients to ensure antibiotics will be an effective treatment in the years to come?

If we expect to continue having this resource available for our children and grandchildren, we need to seriously reconsider every use and be sure it is an appropriate one. Most uses are not justified, especially in the case of ear infections. It has been the policy of the AAP for over a decade to use the "wait and see" approach with ear infections. This approach relies on the research stating that ear infections typically clear up on their own and antibiotics can increase the recurrence of infections by 5-7 times. While I completely understand the need and helpless feeling as a mom to "do something" I want to be sure that what I am doing is actually beneficial, not harmful or prolonging my child's discomfort.

In short, to prevent this overuse and potential loss of one of our most valuable medical tools, we can borrow the statement offered by respected pediatrician Dr. Greene, "If there is any way to safely help her feel better without antibiotics, that is what I would prefer." By this simple statement, parents can make clear their intentions to the doctor and the two can work together to be sure antibiotics are only used when indicated. This statement also removes the pressure to prescribe from the physician.

Obviously, natural alternatives to antibiotics exist and are often effective and even safer ways to treat infections. Ear infections can be treated with massage and osteopathic manipulation techniques, and probiotics (beneficial "friendly" bacteria) can be added to compliment both natural therapies and traditional antibiotic treatments.

Appendix Two: Herbs to Avoid During Pregnancy and Breastfeeding

As I have mentioned throughout this book, there are many herbs that should not be taken during a pregnancy or while breastfeeding. While this list is far from exhaustive, it covers many of the most commonly used herbs that need to be avoided during pregnancy or lactation. The absence of an herb fro this list does not ensure safety for the pregnant or breastfeeding woman, so be sure to always check with an herbalist or care provider with experience in herbal medicine before medicating with herbs during these special times.

Apricot seeds
Arnica
Ashwagandha
Barberry
Bitter almond
Black walnut
Blue cohosh
Boneset
Borage
Buchu
Bugleweed
Castor oil
Comfrey root
Devil's claw
Elecampane
Ephedra (ma huang)
Goldenseal
Gymnema
Horsetail
Kava kava
Lobelia
Oregon grape root
Pennyroyal
Rue
Sassafras
Star anise
Vetiver
Wild cherry

Index

I

J

K

L

M

About The Author

Jessie Hawkins, MH founded Vintage Remedies to answer the growing need of women and mothers everywhere to have a reliable source to turn to for answers to their natural health questions. What began as a small consulting practice blossomed into multiple written works, an extensive website filled with tips and formulas for natural living and more recently, the Vintage Remedies School of Natural Health, which educates individuals throughout the world about the safe and effective use of herbal remedies and natural health.

When she is not consulting, writing or speaking, Jessie stays busy with her many family duties and her home church, Grace Fellowship, PCA. Jessie is a homeschooling mommy, with three children so far, and one more to join the family by way of adoption from Ethiopia. She lives in a Nashville suburb with her husband Matthew and their children.

Other Works by Jessie:

Vintage Remedies Family Herbalist Course, 2007
The Kitchen Herbal with Thistle Publications, 2007
Herbal Crafts with Silverleaf Press, 2008
Lavender with Silverleaf Press, 2008
Vintage Remedies Master Herbalist Course, 2008
Organic Gifts with Thistle Publications, 2008
Herbal Spa with Thistle Publications, 2009